Food Safety and Inspec

CW00685168

The process of food inspection relies on an inspector's understanding of the intrinsic hazards associated with individual foods. Whereas spoilage can usually be determined through a simple organoleptic assessment, the judgment of whether a food is fit for human consumption requires an evaluation of health hazards, many of which may not be apparent through physical assessment. Instead the inspector must analyse and integrate scientific and handling information to evaluate the potential health risk. Adulteration of foods is also becoming an increasing problem, and the complexity of the food supply chain requires an understanding of risk points to allow targeted inspection and assessment.

Food Safety and Inspection: An Introduction focuses on food categories and describes common hazards associated with each, using published peer-reviewed research to explain and evaluate the health risk. It is a practical textbook designed to support the role of food inspection in a modern food industry. There are seven chapters looking at specific aspects of food safety, including a chapter on fraud and adulteration.

This book summarises relevant published research to provide a scientific context for specific food safety issues, and is an essential read for anyone interested in becoming a food inspector.

Madeleine Smith retrained as an Environmental Health Officer in 1993, being awarded the Ronald Williams silver medal before working as an inspector with Birmingham City Council. In 2000 she joined the University of Birmingham, UK, where she developed the food safety provision and now heads the Food Safety Group.

'A practical and user-friendly guide that will appeal to both practitioners and students.'

—*Dr Ajay Patel*, Senior Lecturer in Food Law and Regulation,
Manchester Metropolitan University, UK

'From food parasites to food fraud, this book is an unrivalled source of scientific and peer-reviewed information on food safety and authenticity. Essential reading for anyone wanting a comprehensive understanding of the current risks and controls.'

—*John Barnes*, Former Head of Local Delivery,
Food Standards Agency

Food Safety and Inspection

An Introduction

Madeleine Smith

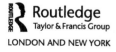

Routledge
Taylor & Francis Group

LONDON AND NEW YORK

First published 2019
by Routledge
2 Park Square, Milton Park, Abingdon, Oxon OX14 4RN

and by Routledge
711 Third Avenue, New York, NY 10017

*Routledge is an imprint of the Taylor & Francis Group, an informa
business*

British Library Cataloguing-in-Publication Data
A catalogue record for this book is available from the British Library

Library of Congress Cataloging-in-Publication Data
Names: Smith, Madeleine (Madeleine P.), author.
Title: Food safety and inspection : an introduction / Madeleine Smith.
Description: Abingdon, Oxon ; New York, NY : Routledge, [2018] |
    Includes bibliographical references and index.
Identifiers: LCCN 2018005265 | ISBN 9780815353539 (hbk) | ISBN
    9780815353546 (pbk) | ISBN 9781351136105 (ebk)
Subjects: LCSH: Food adulteration and inspection.
Classification: LCC TX531 .S6464 2018 | DDC 363.19/264—dc23
LC record available at https://lccn.loc.gov/2018005265

ISBN: 978-0-8153-5353-9 (hbk)
ISBN: 978-0-8153-5354-6 (pbk)
ISBN: 978-1-351-13610-5 (ebk)

Typeset in Times New Roman
by Apex CoVantage, LLC

This book is dedicated to all the people who have
studied food safety at the University of Birmingham.
Thank you for your participation
and questions.

Contents

Figures

Tables

Preface

The idea for this book arose while I was developing course materials to support a module in practical food inspection, which the University of Birmingham, in collaboration with colleagues at Birmingham City Council, has been running since 2008. The main purpose is to provide background information from research publications for some food safety issues. Where possible, I have tried to apply the research findings to practical food inspection, focusing on areas that I would have found interesting or useful when I worked as a local government inspector. My aim was to provide a scientific context for the control of some specific food safety hazards.

The book was written with food safety inspectors in mind, but the information may also be of interest to people working in the food industry, as, in common with local government inspectors, many might not have the time or the opportunity to access the scientific literature themselves. However, there are full reference lists at the end of each chapter should readers wish to read the original research papers.

I have assumed readers will possess the basic knowledge of food microbiology required to work as a food inspector. Anyone needing a refresher in this area can consult one of the excellent textbooks available, such as *Food Microbiology* by Adams, Moss and McClure (2016). I have based the discussion of controls on the food legislation in use in the UK and EU at the time of writing. Although it may not be directly applicable to any readers outside the EU, the standards set under this legislation provide a high level of public health protection and form a good basis for the delivery of controls. Countries with developed food control systems will undoubtedly have similar standards although the names and arrangements of the regulations will obviously be specific to that country.

There are always unanswered questions, and some of the chapters end with such issues, for example, the possible effect of masked mycotoxins in Chapter 5. However, I hope that my summaries and application of what has been published so far by the research scientists will be of some use to food specialists in evaluating food safety risks and determining appropriate controls.

Madeleine Smith

Acknowledgments

I would like to thank the Food Safety Group at University of Birmingham, especially Gill Burrows, course administrator extraordinaire, for their continual help and enthusiasm. I am very grateful to Jim Nettleship for his invaluable advice and practical input on this book. Thanks are also due to my friends and colleagues at Birmingham City Council, where I first learned about inspecting food.

Abbreviations

ACMSF	Advisory Committee on the Microbiological Safety of Food
APHA	Animal and Plant Health Agency (UK)
a_w	Water activity
BRC	British Retail Consortium
BSI	British Standards Institute
CCP	Critical Control Point
Codex Alimentarius	International standards published by the FAO /WHO
DEFRA	Department of Environment Food and Rural Affairs (UK)
DPI	Designated Point of Import
EC	European Commission
ECDC	European Centre for Disease Prevention and Control
EFSA	European Food Safety Authority
Eh	Redox potential
EU	European Union
FAO	Food and Agriculture Organisation (UN)
FDA	Food and Drugs Administration (USA)
FDF	Food and Drink Federation (UK)
FSA	Food Standards Agency (UK)
GAP	Good Agricultural Practice
HACCP	Hazard Analysis Critical Control Points
HTST	High Temperature Short Time
HUS	Haemolytic Uremic Syndrome
IARC	International Agency for Research on Cancer
IID	Infectious Intestinal Disease
MAP	Modified Atmosphere Packing
PFGE	Pulsed Field Gel Electrophoresis
PNOAO	Products not of animal origin
POA	Products of animal origin
RASFF	Rapid Alert System for Food and Feed
SSA	Seasoning and Spices Association (UK)
WHO	World Health Organization

1   Parasites associated with fish

A parasite is defined as an organism that lives in or on another organism, deriving shelter and/or nutrition from the host. Typically the parasite receives benefit from the relationship, but the host does not. The host is usually disadvantaged by the relationship, although it is not normally in the interests of the parasite to affect the host so badly that the host dies prematurely. Parasites associated with fish are mainly worms. There are two important phyla of worms that contain parasitic members. These are the flatworms (Platyhelminthes) and the roundworms (Nematoda).

Platyhelminthes (flatworms)

There are three classes of flatworms but only two are parasitic: the trematodes (liver flukes) and cestodes (tapeworms). Platyhelminth worms are ideally adapted to a parasitic life style as they are often small flattened creatures with fairly simple organ systems. They have only one opening to the digestive tract (or in the case of tapeworms, no digestive tract at all) and some rely on nutrients passing across the body wall or tegument. The body wall is also the site where gaseous exchange occurs, there being no equivalent of a lung. Nitrogenous waste is also passed across the tegument. Species that are endoparasitic (all those described here) are facultative anaerobes since the oxygen supply within a host's organ systems will be limited.

Both classes have marine and freshwater representatives and typically have quite complex life cycles. Unlike meat, there is not a universal system of inspection that can control the hazard of parasites in fish prior to placing on the market. This means that in some parts of the world they are a significant source of morbidity.

Trematoda (liver flukes)

As their common name implies, the adult form of this class inhabits the liver of the primary host. The primary host is typically a mammal, and the adult parasite infests the host's bile ducts, causing thickening, inflammation and blockage. The adult worm is small (usually only a couple of centimetres long) and flattened.

Many have hooks around the edge of the body to assist their movement through the bile ducts of the host liver. This action contributes to the irritation and discomfort associated with the infestation. Substantial numbers of the parasite can build up in a host, causing blockages of the bile ducts.

The parasites have multi-stage life cycles involving intermediate hosts. The intermediate hosts contain the juvenile or intermediate stages of the worm. The primary host (a vertebrate) contains the adult. Trematodes are hermaphrodites. Eggs from the adults are deposited into water and a free-swimming larva known as a miracidium develops. This penetrates the epidermis of the intermediate host and goes through various developmental stages there, typically in the digestive gland. The developed larva (cercaria) will leave the host via the digestive system and is usually eaten by a second intermediate host, where it encysts to form what is known as the metacercaria. The life cycle is completed when the second intermediate host is eaten (raw) by the primary host. The metacercaria then excysts and migrates to its target spot, where it matures into an adult worm.

There are an estimated 70 species of trematodes that affect humans via food sources (WHO 2002) and a number of these species of liver fluke use fish as one of their intermediate hosts. They include *Clonorchis sinensis* (Chinese liver fluke) and *Opisthorcis felineus* (Siberian fluke). *Clonorchis sinensis* is endemic in China, Japan, Korea and Taiwan (Kaewpitoon *et al.* 2008). In Thailand *O. viverrini* is the native parasite, and in Eastern Europe it is *O. felineus* (Kaewpitoon *et al.* 2008). All have very similar life cycles involving two intermediate hosts (a fish and a mollusc) with a mammal (human) as a primary host. The mature worms can be very long-lived, surviving in the bile ducts for up to ten years in some cases. The life cycle of a typical trematode *Clonorchis sinensis* is shown as an example (Figure 1.1).

The key issue is that the primary host (the mammal) must eat the second intermediate host (the fish) raw. Cooking destroys the metacercaria larva and no infection will occur. Metacercariae survive and remain viable in the raw product for a number of hours after the fish dies. This strategy is presumably to maximise the opportunity for infecting the primary host. Freshly killed raw fish are the most dangerous but chilling or freezing can in fact prolong the viability of the larvae. Wiwanitkit *et al.* (2001 and 2002) found that refrigeration and freezing slow the degeneration of the metacercaria to between 5 and 8 hours. They estimate that it may take up to 12 hours after the fish dies for the larvae to fully degenerate under chilled conditions.

Wiwanitkit *et al.* (2002) estimated there were approximately 21 million cases of human infection by liver flukes worldwide, although this is difficult to assess accurately. There is a high prevalence of trematode parasites in South East Asia, mainly due to the popularity of eating raw fish, especially very freshly killed fish. A survey of 79 fish in a Thai reservoir found that a substantial number (16 fish or 20%) were infected with active metacercariae (Wiwanitkit *et al.* 2001). Infection with liver flukes will normally cause at least abdominal pain and indigestion, and often more serious symptoms such as diarrhoea; jaundice; gastrointestinal

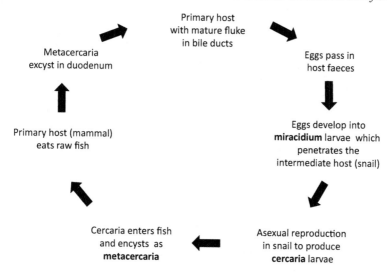

Figure 1.1 Life cycle of *Clonorchis sinensis*

bleeding; formation of gallstones; enlarged gall bladder; weakness and weight loss; portal hypertension; ascites; inflammation and hyperplasia of the biliary epithelium leading to deposition of fibrous tissue. Anorexia has also been reported and, in heavy infections of *Clonorchis sinensis,* there may be an invasion of the pancreatic duct (WHO 2002). Faecal screening can be carried out, but the organism may be difficult to detect in new cases or where infestation is light (WHO 2002). Treatment can be carried out using antihelminths such as praziquantel (Wiwanitkit *et al.* 2001, 2002).

Control

The best control is the thorough cooking of all fish prior to eating. However, raw fish is a traditional delicacy in many parts of the world and is increasingly popular in the UK and USA (Terramocci *et al.* 2001). As mentioned already, the larvae remain infective for some hours after the fish is killed, and chilling prolongs the viability. Fan (1998) found viable metacercariae after freezing the infested fish for up to seven days at -20°C. In this experiment 100% of the laboratory rats used for testing were found to be infected by the pre-frozen larvae. In a similar experiment where the fish were frozen for 18 days at -12°C, the same researcher found a 75% infection rate in rabbits. Under experimental conditions, drying (air) and/ or marinating in 5% vinegar or 5% NaCl appear to speed up the destruction of the metacercariae. After three hours at room temperature, the larvae had degenerated (Wiwanitkit *et al.* 2002). This suggests that the traditional condiments of salty fermented sauces (soy sauce or fish sauce) and vinegar, which often act as a marinade or accompany raw fish dishes, might provide a hurdle, but are not on their own sufficient to destroy the larvae if the fish is to be eaten very fresh. It should also be noted that there is conflicting evidence. Fan (1998) found viable and infective larvae after salting fish at room temperature for up to seven days. He used a salt concentration of 3g salt /10g fish, which seems extremely high compared to the work reported by Wiwanitkit *et al.* (2002). However, Fan reports that larvae still infected 100% of the laboratory rats used to test viability after this treatment.

The disposal of human sewage is another issue for the life cycle of these liver flukes. The eggs from the adult trematode are passed in the faeces of the mammalian (human) host. If the human and animal faeces are treated and controlled, the life cycle of this parasite will be interrupted. However, in some countries raw human sewage is still allowed to contaminate water courses. In fact, according to the WHO report (2002), many rural households have a pool or pond in which to raise fish for their own (or others') consumption. Householders deliberately add human and animal excrement to the pool as a fertiliser. The report describes the 'widespread use of latrines constructed on stilts directly over fishponds or beside them' and suggests this is a major source of contamination with regard to trematode infection. It is difficult to disagree with this conclusion.

Destruction of snails has also been suggested by the WHO as a possible control measure. However, as the larval stages inhabit several species of snail (and several species of fish) (Kaewpitoon *et al.* 2008), correct disposal of human sewage would probably be a more effective option – and would also interrupt the transmission of many other diseases passed via the faecal-oral route, in addition to limiting trematode infections.

Cestoda (tapeworms)

The cestodes are tapeworms, and there are several species where the primary host is a mammal. The intermediate hosts are usually a crustacean and a fish. As with the trematodes, the fish (second intermediate host) must be eaten raw by the primary host (mammal) for infection to occur. *Diphyllobothrium latum* is a well-reported tapeworm that uses fresh water crustacean and fish as intermediate hosts.

Diplogonoporus grandis is also reported as causing morbidity, but less appears to be known about this organism. The life cycle of *Diphyllobothrium latum* is shown as a typical example of the group (Figure 1.2).

Diphyllobothrium latum is a long-lived parasite which has been known to inhabit human hosts for up to 20 years. During that time it can grow to significant size in the host's small intestine, for example, 15 meters (Raether and Hänel 2003). It is commonly but not exclusively found in cold water fish, and infections have been reported in North and South America, Russia, Japan and Europe (Raether and Hänel 2003, Terramocci *et al.* 2001) as well as warmer countries such as Korea (Lee *et al.* 2001). Given the organism's freshwater distribution, fish with a high risk of transmitting the parasite include pike, perch, ruffe and turbot, as well as the salmonids (Raether and Hänel 2003, Terramocci *et al.* 2001, Lee *et al.* 2001). There are marine species in this group as well. Kino *et al.* (2002) reported 46 cases of *Diplogonoporus grandis* in Japan in 1996, some of which appear to

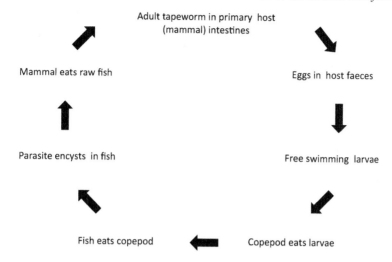

Figure 1.2 Life cycle of *Diphyllobothrium latum*

have been caused by the consumption of raw juvenile anchovies. Other suspected sources include raw tuna and jack mackerel.

Humans who are infected with *D. latum* may show few symptoms. The ripe proglottids pass in the faeces and can be noticed, but there is apparently very little discomfort associated with the process. According to Raether and Hänel (2003), approximately 2% of infected individuals develop pernicious anaemia as a result of the parasite. Kino *et al.* (2002) found symptoms in many of the participants in their study of *Diplogonoporus grandis*. However these were relatively mild, the main symptom being diarrhoea (94.6% of participants). Other symptoms included abdominal pain, fever and vomiting and, in one case, perhaps unsurprisingly, 'a strange abdominal feeling'. Patients became aware of the infection when the worms spontaneously evacuated. The patients then presented themselves for medical treatment. Similarly in the incidents reported by Terramocci *et al.* (2001) of *D. latum* infections in Italy, the victims were either asymptomatic or displayed mainly diarrhoea and/or abdominal pain.

As with trematode infestation, the distribution of illness relates to the culture of eating raw fish. Lee *et al.* (2001) report two cases of *D. latum* in Korea from eating raw cherry salmon and Terramocci *et al.* (2001) report six cases of D. *latum* around Lake Como, Italy, between September 1998 and December 1999 from raw perch. Other more recent incidents can be found in the literature from various parts of the world and researchers suggest that increasing numbers are coming to the attention of medical staff. Part of this might be due to the development of aquaculture which can introduce a species to areas where it was previously unknown. This appears to have happened in South America where incidents of the disease are reported in both Brazil and Chile, although the parasite is not native in Brazil (Cabello 2007). It is suggested that the escape of salmonids from aquaculture tanks has provided the opportunity for the parasite to infect native fish and the practice of exporting fish to Brazil has allowed the parasite to infect people in places where it is not endemic. The other practice that is increasing the incidence of this parasite is the increase in the popularity of raw fish dishes, such as sushi, in areas where it was not traditional (Terramocci *et al.* 2001).

Control

As with trematode parasites, the best control is to cook fish before eating. This destroys the encysted larvae. One of the six patients in Italy described by Terramocci *et al.* (2001) claimed to have eaten smoked rather than raw fish. Torres *et al.* (1989) also suggest that smoked fish can be a source of infection. Unfortunately, unlike the trematodes, there is little recent published experimental data giving any information about the longevity of the encysted larvae or their resistance to heat, cold, acid or salt. It does not appear from the notified cases that cold smoking will kill the larva, but the temperatures used were not reported. It is possible that freezing and/or salting can have a detrimental effect on viability, but there is no published data to indicate appropriate temperatures, times or concentrations. Given the larvae's ability to survive gastric juices, they are likely to have some survival mechanism to withstand low pH. The conclusion must be that only thorough cooking can be confirmed as an effective control. Further research might identify a safe freezing time/temperature regime that would render raw or cold smoked fish safe to eat, but at the moment this information is not available.

Nematoda (roundworms)

Nematodes are a different phylum from the flatworms. They have a more complex body structure and, as their common name implies, are round in cross section rather than flat. The group is a very large one, and not all the members are parasitic. Many species live independent lives in soil and water and are not in any way harmful to humans. The parasitic species are much less impressive to look at than the flatworms – they do not have specialised suckers or hooks to insert into their victims, and they tend not to grow very large. They are just small, slim, pale or orange/brown worms that are pointed at both ends. They are radially symmetric and have a complex cuticle or covering that is protective. The juveniles are very similar to the adults but smaller and with immature or missing organ systems. The two species that form a food safety hazard with respect to fish are:

- *Pseudoterranova decipiens* – codworm
- *Anasakis simplex* – herring worm.

A related species, *Anisakis pegreffi*, also appears to have pathogenic potential (Jeon and Kim 2015). There are fewer reports of this species causing human infection, but that could be due to the difficulty in speciating the larval forms. Modern molecular methods allow more accurate identification of species than in the past, so it is possible that some of the cases which were said to be caused by *Anasakis simplex* could have been the result of infection by *Anisakis pegreffi*.

Pseudoterranova decipiens is found in cod, as its common name suggests, but has also been identified in other fish including hake, mackerel, red conger eel, halibut and arctic smelt. It is approximately 25mm long, orange/brown or pale in colour. *Anasakis simplex* is very similar and has been found in whiting, herrings, mackerel, salmon, cod, halibut, sardines and squid. It is reported to be smaller than *Pseudoterranova decipiens,* but the differences need an expert to determine.

The primary host of both worms are marine mammals – seals for *Pseudoterranova decipiens* and whales, porpoise, dolphins for *Anasakis simplex*. Humans can also be affected if they consume raw fish infected with the juvenile stages. The life cycle for *Pseudoterranova decipiens* is shown in Figure 1.3. The life cycle for *Anasakis simplex* is very similar although the preferred species of intermediate and primary hosts are slightly different. In both species, the eggs are passed into the sea water in the faeces of the primary host. In the salt water they undergo a maturation stage before developing into juveniles which are eaten by the first intermediate host – krill or other crustacea. Some development occurs inside the crustacean and when the crustacean is eaten by a fish or squid, the larvae burrow out into the peritoneal cavity of the fish. They may encapsulate there or progress onto the viscera or muscles. When the primary host eats the fish (raw) the larvae develop into adults in the host digestive system. Although the primary risk is associated with the ingestion of raw vertebrate fish, for example herring, Shweiki *et al.* (2014) report a case of small bowel obstruction by *Anasakis simplex* which was acquired by eating raw clams.

Pseudoterranova decipiens mainly restricts itself to the stomach in human hosts. It can penetrate the gastric tissue but apparently tends not to be as invasive

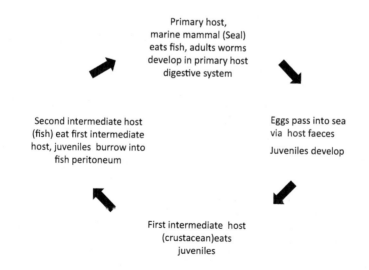

Figure 1.3 Life cycle of *Pseudoterranova decipiens*

as *Anisakis simplex* (Mercado *et al.* 2001). Infection can result in nausea, pharyngeal or abdominal pain and coughing. Frequently there is natural elimination of the worm between 36 hours and 14 days after ingestion of raw fish (by expectoration). Invasion into the soft tissues of the host is rare but has been reported (Sakanari and McKerrow 1989; Shimamura *et al.* 2016). Reports of cases occur wherever raw fish is eaten – for example Mercado *et al.* (2001) identify seven cases between 1997–1999 in Chile, Yu *et al.* (2001) report a case in Korea in 1994 and Shimamura *et al.* (2016) describe cases in Canada.

Anisakis simplex rarely reaches full maturity in humans but can cause illness and occasionally (in 0.4% of cases) can invade the gastric mucosa and migrate to other sites (Takabe *et al.* 1998; Shweiki *et al.* 2014). There are two forms of anisakidosis: gastric or intestinal (Shimamura *et al.* 2016; Sakanari *et al.* 1989). The majority of infections are gastric (97%) and similar to those described for *Pseudoterranova decipiens*. The disease tends to be self-limiting with nausea and vomiting 2–5 hours after ingestion. Eventually the worm is coughed up by the (probably slightly surprised) host and eliminated. However those cases with intestinal anisakidosis tend to be more serious. There can be an allergic reaction and mucosal swelling (several days after ingestion) with potential developments such as strangulating intestinal obstruction (Takabe *et al.* 1998), intestinal thickening, damage, oedema and abscess (Couture *et al.* 2003). Surgery is usually required to remove the worms and to repair damage as anti-helminths appear ineffective.

Incidence

Jeon and Kim (2015) estimate that approximately 2,000 cases of *Anisakis* infection are identified each year, with 90% being reported in Japan. Improved diagnostic techniques might result in increased reports from other parts of the world. There is a high incidence of parasitised fish in areas with large marine mammal populations. A five-year survey in Tokyo wholesale market (Takabe *et al.* 1998) identified that 98% of mackerel and 94% of cod had infestations of the final larval stage. Chen and Shih (2015) also report high levels of parasitism (72.8%) in mackerel caught in Taiwanese waters. In a sample of 64 fish from the US NW Coast (salmon and rockfish) all were parasitised – 3,545 larvae were recovered in total (Deardroff and Throm 1988). Sampling carried out in Sardinia in 2013 found that, overall, 39.9 % of the fish were infested. Chub mackerel (*Scomber colias*) had the highest level of infestation (100% of the sample) but hake (*Merluccius merluccius*) was also heavily parasitised (Casti *et al.* 2017). The larvae will accumulate during the life time of the fish, so older (larger) fish are more heavily contaminated than younger (smaller) ones (Young 1972; Casti *et al.* 2017). A recent Food Standards Agency survey confirms this, stating that in the fish surveyed, the numbers of parasites increased with the size for the fish. The survey tested fish caught in the North Sea and reported that 50.3% of the cod sampled were positive for *Anisakis simplex* while 37.9% contained *Pseudoterranova decipiens* (Petrie *et al.* n.d.). Monkfish, herring and mackerel were also sampled, and the parasitism ranged from 22.9% to 36% of fish caught. However, the incidence is patchy and thought to be related to the presence of cetaceans and other marine mammals. A survey of 1,050 anchovies and 750 sardines in the Ligurian Sea demonstrated a much lower incidence of between 0 (sardines) and 0.8% (anchovies) (Serracca *et al.* 2014) while the same species surveyed in the North Adriatic also had a low level of parasitism (0.2–0.5%) (Cavallero *et al.* 2015).

In freshly killed fish, *Anisakis simplex* tends to be found in the viscera of the fish with approximately 3% actually in the flesh (Hauk 1977), often around the belly flaps. *Pseudoterranova decipiens* tends to be found elsewhere in the main musculature or fillets as well as viscera and belly flaps (Young 1972, FSA 2008). However, there is evidence that on the death of the fish, the larvae tend to move from the viscera into the flesh (Hauk 1977) presumably to enhance survival until ingestion by a primary host can occur.

Controls

Many fish species can act as a host to the larval stages of both *Pseudoterranova decipiens* and *Anisakis simplex*, including the cod family, halibut and other flat-fish, mackerel, herring, salmon and squid. Some of these species might be eaten raw, pickled or cold smoked. Hot smoking will kill the larvae as it effectively cooks the product but cold smoking, using temperatures of only 20–30°C, does not. In a study of herring using a commercial smoking kit, temperatures of the product varied between 18–41°C and 26–57°C depending on whether the fish was whole or not. In the former group (18–41°C) the researchers found 87.5% of the larvae still viable after a smoking process of 24 hours (Hauk 1977).

Given that the larvae need to survive the acid of a mammalian stomach, they are quite acid tolerant and are not therefore destroyed by pickling or marinating in vinegar or lemon juice. Sakanari and McKerrow (1989) report that *Anisakis* larvae can survive 51 days in vinegar. Adams *et al.* (1997) report work done by Smith and Wootten in 1978 where a typical pickling solution of 6% salt and 4% acid was used to test viability. It was found that 70 days were required to destroy the parasites. Even with a stronger solution of 15% salt and 7% acid, 3% of the worms were alive after 30 days. Roll mop herrings and other uncooked, pickled fish have the potential to transmit these parasites because the treatment is not sufficient to guarantee destruction of all larvae in the fish.

Freezing does seem to destroy the larvae provided the time and temperature is sufficiently extreme. Satisfactory freezing regimes appear to be 15 hours at −35°C (Deardorff and Throm 1988; FDA 2011) or seven days at −20°C (Adams *et al.* 1997, FDA 2011). Cold smoked products like smoked salmon are frequently frozen after smoking to allow thin slicing and provided this process reaches the required temperatures for the requisite amount of time, the product should be safe. Fish to be pickled should be frozen before processing. This freezing stage can be a Critical Control Point to control nematode transmission.

Partial Controls

Immediate evisceration of fish will help to reduce infestation of the flesh as this will prevent the migration of the nematode larvae into the main fillets. The belly flap, which is often the most heavily parasitised (Young 1972) can also be discarded as a partial control. Some papers suggest candling could be a way of detecting parasite infection. However the effectiveness of this control depends on a number of variables such as the type of fish, thickness of fillet and skill of the operator. It can detect 53–79% of infected fillets (Adams *et al.* 1997) but is very time consuming and probably not practical in an industrial context.

Unusable controls

Irradiation has been considered as a possible control measure but at sufficiently high levels to kill the parasite, the taste and texture of the fish are apparently affected (Adams *et al.* 1997). A similar problem exists with the use of High Hydrostatic Pressure treatment. Treatment of 30 seconds at 414MPa and 180 seconds at 207MPa killed 100% of larvae but caused colour change in the fish, especially salmon (Dong *et al.* 2003), rendering it unsuitable for use.

Legislation and inspection

Regulation EC 853/2004, annex III, section VIII, chapter V (D) requires that food business operators should carry out a visual inspection of fishery products and not place parasitised products on the market. Visual inspections will probably be insufficient to ensure removal of all risk, so Regulation EC 852/2004, annex II, chapter IX(1) makes it a prohibition for food business operators to accept raw materials contaminated with parasites to such an extent that processing would not ensure safety. Thorough cooking will destroy the parasites of all the aforementioned species and is a Critical Control Point, although consumers who have been unfortunate enough to find cooked nematodes in their fish suppers are rarely very enthusiastic, in spite of assurances that no health risk exists. The significant health risk is associated with eating raw fish, including cold smoked or pickled products such as smoked salmon and rollmops. Regulation EC 853/2004, annex III, section VIII, chapter III (D)(1) requires fish which is to be eaten raw or cold smoked under 60°C to be frozen at -20°C for a minimum of 24 hours or -35°C for a minimum of 15 hours. Herring, mackerel, sprat, wild salmon and marinated/salted fish are listed specifically as being covered by this requirement, and documentation confirming the freezing process should accompany the products when placed on the market. It is worth noting that the published research suggests that the fish should spend longer than one day at sub-zero temperatures to ensure destruction of the parasites described in this chapter (Deardorff and Throm 1988; FDA 2001; Adams *et al.* 1997, Fan 1998). The minimum legal requirement according to Regulation EC 853/2004 might not be adequate for complete safety but will reduce the risk.

There is an exemption under Regulation EC 853/2004, annex III, section VIII, chapter III (D)(2) from the need to freeze fish if the producer can confirm (using epidemiological data) that the fish originates from waters that do not have a parasite risk and the competent authority accepts and authorises this. Surveys carried out in the Ligurian Sea and North Adriatic (Serrecca *et al.* 2014 and Cavallero *et al.* 2015) provide sampling evidence which can support such claims for certain species. Farmed fish are usually fed controlled food (pellets) which are not contaminated with the parasitic juveniles or larvae, and this can help reduce the hazard by interrupting the natural life cycle of the parasite. A study carried out by the Institute of Aquaculture, University of Stirling and funded by the Food Standards Agency considered 720 samples of farmed Scottish salmon over a six-month period. None of the samples contained any anisakid larvae (Wootten *et al.* 2010). This supports the conclusion that farmed salmon do not pose any significant risk of parasitism. As a consequence of this and other research, EFSA has reviewed the guidance on the use of farmed fish for raw products such as sushi. Provided the farms meet the requirements listed in the guidance with regard to feeding and protection from natural sources, the fish may be placed on the market for consumption raw or cold smoked without the need to freeze (EFSA 2011, FSA 2012). Food business operators handling fish products intended for human consumption that are either raw, cold smoked, marinated or salted should be able to demonstrate compliance with one or other of these controls. This should include documentary evidence of the freezing process or traceability documents relating to an approved supplier compliant with the EFSA guidance.

References

Adams, A., K. Murrell and J.H. Cross (1997); Parasites of fish and risks to public health; *Revue scientifique et technique (International Office of Epizootics)* 16(2), 652–660

Cabello, F. (2007); Salmon aquaculture and transmission of the fish tapeworm; *Emerging Infectious Diseases* 13(1):169–173

Casti, D., C. Scarano, M. Piras, P. Merella, S. Muglia, F. Piras, G. Garippa, C. Spanu and E. De Santis (2017); Occurrence of nematodes of the genus *Anisakis* in Mediterranean and Atlantic fish marketed in Sardinia; *Italian Journal of Food Safety* 6:6185

Cavallero, S., C. Magnabosco, M. Civettini, L. Boffo, G. Mingarelli, P. Buratti, O. Giovanardi, C.M. Fortuna, G. Arcangeli (2015); Survey of *Anisakis* sp. and *Hysterothylacium* sp. in sardines and anchovies from the North Adriatic Sea; *International Journal of Food Microbiology* 200(2015):18–21

Chen, H-Y. and H-H. Shih (2015); Occurrence and prevalence of fish-borne *Anisakis* larvae in the spotted mackerel *Scomber australasicus* from Taiwanese waters; *Acta Tropica* 145(2015): 61–67

Couture, C., L. Measures, J. Gagnon and C. Desblens (2003); Human intestinal anisakiosis due to consumption of raw salmon; *American Journal of Surgical Pathology* 27(8):1167–1172

Deardroff, T.L. and R. Throm (1988); Commercial blast freezing of third stage *Anisakis simplex* larvae encapsulated in salmon and rockfish; *Journal of Parasitic Diseases* 74(4):600–603

Dong, F.M., A.R. Cook and R.P. Herwig (2003); High hydrostatic pressure treatment of finfish to inactivate *Anisakis simplex*; *Journal of Food Protection* 66(10):1924–1926

EFSA (2011); Guidance on viable parasites in fishery products that may represent a risk to the health of the consumer: Endorsed 16 November 2011 by the Standing Committee on the Food Chain; https://ec.europa.eu/food/sites/food/files/safety/docs/biosafety_fh_eu_food_establishments-20111214_scfcah_guidance_parasites_en.pdf accessed November 2017

Fan, P.C. (1998); Viability of metacercariae of *Clonorchis sinensis* in frozen or salted freshwater fish; *International Journal for Parasitology* 28:603–5

Food and Drugs Administration (2001); Fish and fisheries products hazards and controls guidance; http://www.cfsan.fda.gov/~comm/haccp4.html accessed November 2008

Food and Drugs Administration (2011); Fish and fisheries products hazards and controls guidance; 4th edition, chapter 5; https://www.fda.gov/downloads/food/guidanceregulation/ucm251970.pdf accessed November 2017

Food Standards Agency (2008); A survey of *Anisakis* and *Pseudoterranova* in Scottish fisheries and the efficacy of current detection methods; http://www.food.gov.uk/science/research/researchinfo/devolvedadmins/scotlandresearch/scotlandresearch/ScotlandProjectList/s14008/#results accessed November 2008

Food Standards Agency (2012); Fish freezing requirements relaxed; http://www.food.gov.uk/news-updates/news/2012/jul/fishfreeze accessed October 2012

Hauk, A.K. (1977); Occurrence and survival of the larval nematode *Anisakis* sp in the flesh of fresh, frozen, brined and smoked Pacific herring, *Clupea harengus pallasi*; *Journal of Parasitology* 63(3):515–519

Jeon, C-H. and J-H. Kim (2015); Pathogenic potential of two sibling species, *Anasakis simplex* and *Anisakis pegreffi* (Nematoda: Anisakidae): *In Vitro* and *In Vivo* studies; *BioMed Research International* 2015; doi:10.1155/2015/983656

Kaewpitoon, N., S.J. Kaewpitoon and P. Pengsaa (2008); Opisthorchiasis in Thailand: Review and current status; *World Journal of Gastroenterology* 14(15):2297–2302

Kino, H., W. Hori, H. Kobayashi, N. Nakamura and K. Nagasawa (2002); A mass occurrence of human infection with *Diplogonoporus Grandis* (Cestoda: Diphyllobothriidae) In Shizuoka Prefecture, Central Japan; *Parasitology International* 51:73–79

Lee, K., H-C. Suhk, K-S. Pai, H-J. Shin, S-Y. Jung, E-T. Han and J-Y. Chai (2001); *Diphyllobothrium latum* infection after eating domestic salmon flesh; *Korean Journal of Parasitology* 39(4): 319–321

Mercado, R., P. Torres, V. Muñoz, W. Apt (2001); Human infection by *Pseudoterranova decipiens* (Nematoda, Anisakidae) in Chile: Report of seven cases; *Memórias do Instituto Oswaldo Cruz* 96(5):653–655

Petrie, A., R. Wootten, D. Bruno, K. MacKenzie and J. Bron (n.d.); A survey of Anisakis and Pseudoterranova in Scottish fisheries and the efficacy of current detection methods; FSAS Project S14008 1st July 2005 to 31st June 2007; http://citeseerx.ist.psu.edu/viewdoc/download?doi=10.1.1.424.1745&rep=rep1&type=pdf accessed March 14 2018

Raether, W. and H. Hänel (2003); Epidemiology, clinical manifestations and diagnosis of zoonotic cestode infections: An update; *Parasitology Research* 91: 412–438

Sakanari, J. and J.H. Mckerrow (1989); *Anisakiasis Clinical Microbiology Reviews* 2(3):278–284

Serracca, L., R. Battistini, I. Rossini, A. Carducci, M. Verani, M. Prearo, L. Tomei, G. De Montis, C. Ercolini (2014); Food safety considerati ons in relation to *Anisakis pegreffi* in anchovies (*Engraulis encrasicolus*) and sardines (*Sardina pilchardus)* fished off the Ligurian Coast; *International Journal of Food Microbiology* 190 (2014):79–83

Shimamura Y., N. Muwanwella, S. Chandran, G. Kandel and N. Marcon (2016) Common symptoms from an uncommon infection: Gastrointestinal Anisakiasis. *Canadian Journal of Gastroenterology and Hepatology 2016*; doi:10.1155/2016/5176502

Shweiki, E., D. Rittenhouse, J. Ochoa, V. Punja, M. Zubair and J. Balif (2014) Acute small-bowel obstruction from intestinal Anisakiasis after the ingestion of raw clams; documenting a new method of marine-to-human parasitic transmission; *Open Forum Infectious Diseases* 1(2); doi:v10.1093/ofid/ofu087

Takabe, K., S. Ohki, O. Kunihiro, T. Sakashita, I. Endo, Y.Ichikawa, H. Sekido, T. Amano, Y. Nakatani, K. Suzuki, H. Shimada (1998); Anisakidosis: A cause of intestinal obstruction from eating sushi; *American Journal of Gastroenterology* 93:1172–1173

Terramocci, R., L. Pagani, P. Brunati, S. Gatti, A. Bernuzzi and M. Scaglia (2001); Reappearance of human diphyllobothriasis in a limited area of Lake Como, Italy; *Infection* 29(2):93–95

Torres P., R. Franjola, J. Pérez, S. Auad, F. Uherek, J.C. Miranda, L. Flores, J. Riquelme, S. Salazar, C. Hermosilla (1989); Epidemiology of diphyllobothriasis in the Valdivia River basin, Chile; *Revista de Saúde Pública* 23(1):45–57 [abstract only, article in Spanish]

WHO (2002); Joint WHO/FAO Workshop on foodborne trematode infections in Asia; Report Series Number: RS/2002/GE/40(VTN)

Wiwanitkit, V., S. Nithiuthai, J. Suwansaksri; C. Chongboonprasert, K. Tangwattakanont (2001); Survival of heterophyid metacercariae in uncooked Thai fish dishes; *Annals of Tropical Medicine and Parasitology* 95(7):725–727

Wiwanitkit, V., S. Nithiuthai and J. Suwansaksri (2002); Motility of minute intestinal fluke, *Haplorchinae* spp, Metacercariae in fish dishes prepared by different uncooked methods; *Medscape General Medicine* 4(1)

Wootten, R., G. Yoon and J. Bron (2010); A Survey of anisakid nematodes in Scottish farmed salmon; FSA Project S14008 http://webarchive.nationalarchives.gov.uk/20130410130454/ http://www.food.gov.uk/science/research/devolvedadmins/scotlandresearch/scotlandre search/ScotlandProjectList/S14008ext/ [summary only available after 2013]

Young, P.C. (1972); The relationship between the presence of larval anisakine nematodes in cod and marine mammals in British home waters; *Journal of Applied Ecology* 9:459–485

Yu, J.R., M. Seo, Y. Kim, M. Oh, W. Sohn (2001); A human case of gastric infection by *Pseudoterranova decipiens* larva; *The Korean Journal of Parasitology* 39(2):193–196

2 Shellfish

The word shellfish describes marine and fresh water invertebrates such as lobsters or mussels which may be used as foodstuffs. There is no legal definition of shellfish, but the term is generally used to include the Crustacea (crabs, lobsters, prawns and shrimps) and the Mollusca (bivalves, gastropods and cephalopods).

Shellfish are biologically very diverse, including two different phyla and many classes of animal. This means they exhibit a number of different feeding strategies. Some of these feeding strategies create the potential for food safety hazards, especially when coupled with the normal methods of cooking associated with the group.

Crustacea

Crustacea are omnivores, and many are also scavengers. Food is grasped by the claws and passed onto the mouthparts for tearing and ingestion. Nearly all the commercially important crustaceans live on the sea floor, and although they can swim for short distances, their heavy shell makes them cumbersome and inefficient. Being in the same phylum as insects, they have jointed feet which can be used effectively for walking. Prawns and shrimps typically live on sandy substrates in 5–30 meters of water. Crabs and lobsters are also shallow water dwellers but can be found on rocky as well as sandy sea beds. The Crustacea have segmented bodies divided into a head, thorax (abdomen) and tail. The tails are very muscular and, in shrimps and prawns, are the part used for human consumption. The tail in lobsters is also very meaty and muscular and is used for human consumption, along with the claws. Crabs have meaty claws, which provide white meat, and some muscles in the main shell (thorax) which provide the brown meat. The digestive organs, glands and other internal body parts are discarded with the shell. This means that the parts of the animal that might concentrate toxins from its diet are not used for human consumption, making this group quite low risk. The fact that they are boiled before eating also reduces the food safety risk. The main hazard associated with this group is that of cross contamination with pathogenic bacteria post cooking, which is no different from any other ready-to-eat food.

Mollusca

Three classes of molluscs are commonly used for human consumption: bivalves, cephalopods and gastropods. The highest risk of these groups are the bivalves. There are two main reasons for this risk – one is their method of feeding (filter feeding) and the other is the method of cooking (either eaten raw or only lightly cooked).

Bivalvia

Regulation (EC) 853/2004 refers to the lamellibranch molluscs in its definition of bivalves. This group (lamellibranch molluscs) is the biggest group of bivalves and includes oysters, mussels, clams and scallops.

The lamellibranchs are those molluscs that filter feed using specialised gills. The gills are folded, ciliated and mucus producing. Water passes over the gill filaments and plankton in the water get trapped in the mucus. The cilia move the mucus with its trapped nutrients into a section of the gill known as the food groove. The nutrients are moved along these grooves to the mouth where ingestion occurs. This process is selective, and particles can be ejected before ingestion by the mollusc. These rejected particles are known as pseudo faeces. Research suggests that selection is based on a variety of criteria, including but not exclusively particle size. The shape and flexibility of the food particle could be significant in selection (Bougrier *et al.* 1997) and probably also the chemical composition since cockles have been observed to reject particles of low or no nutritive value (Inglesias *et al.* 1996). Chemoreceptors have been identified on the relevant feeding organs (Sidari *et al.* 1998) supporting this idea. Bivalves normally have a variety of plankton available to them and appear to select some species as preferable to others of the same size (Shumway *et al.* 1985).

This habit of filtering food has very significant food safety implications. Bivalves are able to concentrate toxins and pathogens from the seawater because their normal diet includes the naturally occurring phytoplankton, some of which are toxic to humans, as well as particulate matter. This particulate matter can include faecal material containing bacteria and viruses. Unlike the Crustacea where only the muscle meat is eaten, molluscs tend to be ingested whole, so the consumer eats all the digestive tract and associated glands. Scallops are an exception where only the adductor muscle and roe are eaten, but with oysters, mussels and clams, generally the entire organism is swallowed. The risk associated with eating bivalves is further increased by the fact that these organisms are often eaten raw or very lightly cooked. Therefore, even heat-labile toxins or heat sensitive bacteria might not be destroyed.

Toxins

There are a number of algae which contain or produce toxins that are harmful to humans if ingested (see Table 2.1). These toxins can also cause a health hazard

Table 2.1 Maximum permitted toxin levels in Regulation (EC) No 853/2004

Illness	Toxin	Organism	Symptoms
Amnesic Shellfish Poisoning (ASP)	Domoic acid *max 20 mg/kg*	Diatoms including *Nitzschia pungens, Pseudonitzschia australis*	**Acute symptoms:** Vomiting and diarrhoea, confusion, loss of memory, disorientation and even coma. **Long term symptoms:** Permanent neurological damage can occur, particularly cognitive dysfunction and symptoms reminiscent of Alzheimer's disease.
Paralytic Shellfish Poisoning (PSP)	*max 800 µgrams/kg*	Dinoflagellates especially *Gonyaulax* spp.	Neurological symptoms including tingling sensation or numbness around the lips (which can spread to the face and neck) prickly sensation in the fingertips and toes, arms and legs. Headache and dizziness, also incoherent speech, stiffness and non-coordination of limbs, weakness, rapid pulse, respiratory difficulty, salivation or temporary blindness, nausea and vomiting. In the most severe cases, paralysis of respiratory muscles may progress to respiratory arrest and death within 2 to 12 hours after consumption. Mortality rate is 8–15%
Diarrhetic Shellfish Poisoning (DSP)	Okadaic acid, Dinophysistoxin Pectenotoxins *max 160 µgrams/kg total* Yessotoxin *max 3.75 mg/kg* Azaspiracids *max 160 µgrams/kg*	Dinoflagellates especially *Dinophysis, Prorocentrum*	Nausea, vomiting, diarrhoea, abdominal pain, chills, headache and fever. Typically lasts 2–3 hours but can be days

if inhaled or if the water containing the algae is drunk or used for swimming or other water sports. However, the most common way for people to be affected is through the consumption of contaminated molluscs. Algae are normally present in seawater, but their concentration varies. Under certain environmental conditions they can build up to very large numbers, creating visible patches of colour in the sea known as blooms, or sometimes, red tides.

Sampling of mussels carried out under algal bloom conditions shows the mussels preferentially selected *Dinophysis* cells from the water (Sidari *et al.* 1998) causing a build-up of the toxin in the mollusc. How well bivalves concentrate the algae and toxin seems to vary between species. Suzuki and Mitsuya (2001) found the concentration of okadaic acid homologues was higher in mussels than in scallops from the same exposure. This was also found by Reizopoulou *et al.* (2008), indicating that mussels would be a higher risk than scallops grown in the same conditions. There is also variation as to where the toxin is most concentrated in the organs of the bivalve. Generally the toxin levels are highest in the digestive organs. Bauder *et al.* (2001) found the concentration of Diarrhetic Shellfish Poisoning (DSP) toxin in scallops to be highest in the viscera (76% of total body toxin) and lowest in the adductor muscle (<12 % of total body burden). The adductor muscle is the main part of the scallop used for human consumption, so again scallops could be considered a lower risk than mussels where the entire body is eaten. The digestive organs and other parts of scallops are generally discarded, although the roe will be eaten. Maximum levels have been set for the toxins in Regulation (EC) 853/2004 Annex III section VII chapter V (see Table 2.1). Molluscs exceeding these limits are not permitted to be placed on the market for human consumption. The levels also apply to retail sale.

Bacteria and viruses

Illness associated with eating bivalves has been recorded since at least 1894 when a typhoid outbreak in the US was attributed to the consumption of shellfish (Rippey 1994). An outbreak in the UK in 1902 was attributed to oysters (Morabia and Hardy 2005a) and is notable not just for the food vehicle but also for the fact that it is the first known example of an environmental health officer (then called a local government board inspector) using a questionnaire to collate food histories and work out a food association (Morabia and Hardy 2005b). Although a number of historical outbreaks have been attributed to bacterial contamination of bivalves, these have become less common. The implementation of controls on harvesting and on disposal of sewage has significantly reduced their frequency. There are occasional outbreaks associated with bacterial contamination of shellfish, but the main cause of bivalve associated gastrointestinal infection is now considered to be viral rather than bacterial (Rippey 1994, Lees 2000).

The controls that have resulted in this decrease in bacterial gastrointestinal illness include restrictions on where molluscs can be gathered, restrictions on sale and the setting of sampling standards. These requirements can be found in Regulation (EC) 853/2004 annex III section VII and Regulation (EC) 854/2004 annex II.

The legislation lays down standards that must be used to categorise the harvesting areas into one of three options. Molluscs harvested from an area designated class A can be used for human consumption. Molluscs harvested from a class A area should not have more than 230 cfu of *E. coli* per 100g of flesh. Molluscs from an area categorised as class B can only be placed on the market after either treatment in a purification centre or relaying. The legislation specifies a maximum level of *E. coli* (4,600 per 100g flesh) that can be found in these molluscs and gives the detection method to be used (five tube, three dilution MPN). The third category is designated as a class C area, and molluscs collected from such areas must be relayed before placing on the market. The maximum *E. coli* contamination in molluscs from a class C area is 46,000 per 100g flesh (same detection method). Any areas providing higher contamination levels can be closed and harvesting prohibited.

Bacterial contamination levels are not related to viral contamination levels in shellfish (Romalde *et al.* 2002, Lees 2000, Hernroth *et al.* 2002) and the use of *E. coli* or other enteric bacteria to indicate the safety of bivalves is generally considered to have limited value. The shellfish can be clear of bacterial contaminants but still harbour virus particles (Formiga-Cruz *et al.* 2003). Determining the viral contamination in shellfish has proved exceptionally difficult for a number of reasons (Doré et al. 2000, Flannery et al. 2009). One is that human pathogenic viruses are not at all easy to culture – indeed the most common cause of human viral gastroenteritis, norovirus (formerly called SRSV or Norwalk-like virus) was, for some time, considered non-culturable (Lees 2000), thereby limiting research in the area. Gradually some researchers (Straub *et al.* 2007) began to report success in the culture of the norovirus, although it is still not a widespread or easily repeatable process (Polo *et al.* 2015). Historically, methods used to identify viral contamination have been lacking in sensitivity, requiring very large contamination levels for success (e.g. SEM, immunoassay). These methods occasionally identified viral contamination in faecal samples but were unsuitable for use in foods, especially in bivalves where the contamination levels are generally low but still above the apparently small infectious dose required (Lees 2000). A standard method for detection and quantification of norovirus and hepatitis A in food stuffs (ISO/TS 15216–1:2013) has finally been developed based on the reverse transcriptase polymerase chain reaction (RT-PCR). One barrier to its development has been that shellfish extracts proved inhibitory to PCR (Lees 2000), although the ISO/TS 15216–1:2013 technique claims to be appropriate for shellfish. The technique has been tested in European shellfish beds and is currently being considered for adoption as an EU standard technique for testing and monitoring viral contamination in foods (Polo *et al.* 2015, La Rosa *et al.* 2017). However, at the moment, while there are specialist labs which can use the RT-PCR to detect norovirus and/or hepatitis A and E in food samples, there are no requirements for routine sampling and monitoring of bivalves or their water for viral particles in the way bacterial pathogens are controlled.

An additional problem is that the standard depuration methods are based on the elimination of bacteria, and there have been a number of reports of viral outbreaks associated with depurated bivalves, indicating that while the methods may be adequate to clear bacterial contamination, they are insufficient to ensure the elimination of pathogenic viruses (Lees 2000, Schwab *et al.* 1998). Experiments carried out by Schwab *et al.* (1998) using oysters and clams allowed a 24-hour period of bioaccumulation with norovirus (Norwalk-like virus) and *E. coli* and then depuration for up to 48 hours. The results showed that although there was a 95% reduction in the bacterial contamination after 48 hours depuration, there was only a 7% reduction in the viral contamination. Tian *et al.* (2007) provide evidence that the viral particles are able to attach to molecules (type A-like histo-blood antigens) in the bivalve gut. Such attachment could increase the bioaccumulation of the virus particles as well as rendering the depuration process ineffective. Other researchers using bacteriophages as indicators have shown that the clearance of viruses from bivalves appears to be dependent on the initial loading as well as the water temperature. Higher temperatures favour the more rapid removal of viruses, but heavily contaminated shellfish can still test positive after seven days even at high water temperatures such as 18–20°C (Lees 2000). Laing *et al.* (2004) reporting on the DEFRA funded research confirm this and state that at low water temperature such as 8°C bivalves may need more than nine days of depuration to eliminate FRNA bacteriophages when the contamination levels are typical of those found in class B areas. Raising the water temperature to 20°C reduces the required time to four days. In light of this research, the normal depuration procedures of up to 48 hours would appear to be completely inadequate for virus control.

The normal particle size which can be filtered by adult bivalves is 1–20 μm (Heras *et al.* 1994), although some may filter larger particles according to the shellfish species and size (Klumpp *et al.* 1992). Isolated bacteria would figure at the lower end of this size range and so could theoretically be filtered out as individual cells. However bivalves have been shown to be effective at filtering and using particulate organic matter (Klumpp *et al.* 1992, Stirling 1995) and synthetic particles of the relevant size (Heras *et al.* 1994), so it is likely that bacteria and viruses would be filtered as part of a clump of organisms and/or bound in organic matter suspended in the sea water. Bioaccumulation of bacterial and viral particles is rapid with high contamination levels measured within the bivalves after 24 hours exposure to contaminated sea water (Schwab *et al.* 1998; Doré and Lees 1995).

As with the dinoflagelate toxins, pathogenic bacteria and viruses appear to be concentrated in the digestive organs and hepatopancreas of many bivalves (Romalde *et al.* 2002, Hernroth *et al.* 2002), and the levels found in the bivalve can be several times the concentration found in the surrounding sea water (Burkhart and Calci 2000). As previously mentioned, norovirus particles can adhere to the intestinal tissue of oysters, clams and mussels (Tian *et al.* 2007), and viruses become attached chemically to the mucus on the filtration gills, rather than just physically entrapped. This process appears to increase as the levels of salinity decrease (Di Giromano *et al.* 1977) suggesting that estuarine areas or conditions of reduced salinity, such as when large deposits of sewage or fresh water move into an area, will favour the uptake of virus particles by the molluscs from the seawater. The association of viral outbreaks and heavy rainfall is well documented (Lees 2000). This is generally attributed to the increased sewage contamination of the area from flooding, but any reduced salinity might also enhance the bioaccumulation.

Virus particles can adhere to the sediment which the molluscs inhabit. While it is possible that they can acquire the viruses directly from the sediment, it would appear that the main source is from the water above them (Landry *et al.* 1983). Viruses that have been deposited on the sediment can survive for some periods of time and then become re-suspended if the sediment is disturbed, for example by tides or storms. Norovirus has also been detected in plankton (Polo *et al.* 2015). Plankton are a food source for bivalves suggesting an additional route of contamination as well as a possible reservoir of contamination.

Cephalopda

Cephalopods are carnivores. Squid and octopus are active and successful hunters and eat fish and other invertebrates, including bivalves. Cuttlefish also hunt invertebrates but are slower swimmers than squid, confining themselves to the sea floor, whereas squid are pelagic. All three orders use their tentacles to grab prey and a very powerful beak to tear it into pieces for ingestion. Octopuses are powerful enough to open bivalve shells by pulling them apart. All three types of cephalopod can produce ink which is used as a screen to confuse predators and allow escape. The cuttlefish in particular produces substantial quantities which can be used as an ingredient in cooking. Pasta, for example, can have cephalopod ink incorporated into the dough, giving black noodles. There are no particular food safety hazards associated with the cephalopods because their eating habits do not tend to concentrate toxins or pathogens, and they are generally thoroughly cooked before eating. If cooked, cooled and then used in salads, the normal issues of cross contamination in ready-to-eat foods apply.

Gastropoda

Marine gastropods such as abalone, winkles and whelks are not filter feeders. They are mainly herbivorous, scraping algae off rocks using a specialist feeding organ called a radula. Generally the algae eaten by the gastropods do not produce toxins harmful to humans. This group is therefore an intrinsically lower risk than the bivalve molluscs. In addition, the normal cooking method for gastropods is to boil thoroughly which further reduces the food safety risk by eliminating any heat-labile contaminants. As with the crustaceans described previously, the main hazard associated with this group is that of cross contamination with pathogenic bacteria post cooking. However, the rasping 'tongue' or radula can also be used on other invertebrates, for scavenging and for sediment feeding, so gastropods like whelks and abalone are more accurately classed as omnivorous or predatory. Occasionally there have been reports of toxic levels of saxitoxin identified in these organisms (Deeds *et al.* 2008). Saxitoxin is associated with Paralytic

Shellfish Poisoning (PSP). What appears to happen is that the gastropods predate on the toxic bivalves and as a consequence the toxin becomes concentrated in the higher predator as is normal when transferring to another trophic level. Deeds *et al.* (2008) provide a summary of reported incidents and these have occurred in the US, Spain, South Africa and Japan. If a body of water is suffering an algal bloom with such levels of toxin that it is unsafe to eat the bivalves, it would also seem unwise to eat gastropods from the same area.

Other invertebrates

Although echinoderms and tunicates are completely different phyla from the molluscs, they can also be considered as types of filter feeders. For this reason, when placed on the market alive, they are covered by the sections of legislation that apply to live bivalve molluscs. Once cooked or processed they are considered to be fishery products. Echinoderms are the group of invertebrates that include sea urchins and sea cucumbers. Their main characteristic is that they are penta-radially symmetric – that is they have a five-rayed symmetry instead of the bilateral symmetry most other organisms show. Sea urchins are eaten in some Caribbean islands and sea cucumbers (holothurians) are popular in some types of Chinese cooking. Tunicates or sea squirts are not very commonly used as food stuff.

Legislation

According to Regulation (EC) 853/2004, shellfish are classified as either a fishery product or a mollusc according to their phylum or class.

A fishery product is defined as 'all seawater or freshwater animals (except for live bivalve molluscs, live echinoderms, live tunicates and live marine gastropods, and all mammals, reptiles and frogs), whether wild or farmed and including all edible forms, part and products of such animals' (Annex I (3) 3.1 Regulation (EC) No 853/2004).

This means that all the Crustacea (crabs, lobsters, shrimps and prawns) and the cephalopods (squid, octopus and cuttlefish) are fishery products. The molluscs, echinoderms and tunicates are considered to be fishery products once cooked or dead but are identified as a different legal category while still alive. Only the bivalve molluscs have a legal definition. A bivalve mollusc is defined as 'a filter-feeding lamellibranch mollusc' (Annex I. (2) 2.1 Regulation (EC) No 853/2004).

Live echinoderms, live tunicates and live marine gastropods are included in the section of Regulation (EC) 853/2004 covering live bivalve molluscs (Annex III, section VII).

Because the bivalve molluscs have such high intrinsic risk of causing a food borne illness, Regulation (EC) 853/2004, Annex III, section VII lays down requirements that apply to their harvest and placing on the market. It should be noted that some parts of this section also apply to retail sale, for example chapters V (health standards), VI (wrapping and packaging), and point 3 of VII (identification and marking).

References

Bauder, A., A.D. Cembella, V.M. Bricelj and M.A. Quilliam (2001); Uptake and fate of diarrhetic shellfish poisoning toxins from the dinoflagellate *Prorocentrum lima* in the bay scallop *Argopecten irradaens*; *Marine Ecology Progress Series* 213:59–32

Bougrier, S., A.J.S. Hawkins and M. Héral (1997); Preingestive selection of different microalgal mixtures in *Crassostrea gigas* and *Myths edulis*, analysed by flow cytometry; *Aquaculture* 150:123–134

Burkhardt, W. and K.R. Calci (2000); Selective accumulation may account for shellfish-associated viral illness; *Applied and Environmental Microbiology* 66(4):1375–1378

Deeds, J.R., J.H. Landsberg, S.M. Etheridge, G.C. Pitcher and S.W. Longan (2008); Non-traditional vectors for paralytic shellfish poisoning; *Marine Drugs* 6(2):308–48.

Di Girolamo, R., J. Liston and J. Matches (1977); Ionic bonding, the mechanism of viral uptake by shellfish mucus; *Applied and Environmental Microbiology* 33(1):19–25

Doré, W.J. and D.N. Lees (1995); Behavior of Escherichia coli and male-specific bacteriophage in environmentally contaminated bivalve molluscs before and after depuration; *Journal of Applied and Environmental Microbiology* 61:2830–2834

Doré, W., K. Henshilwood and D.N. Lees (2000); Evaluation of F-specific RNA bacteriophage as a candidate human enteric virus indicator for bivalve molluscan shellfish; *Applied and Environmental Microbiology* 66(4):1280–1285

Flannery, J., S. Keaveney and W. Doré (2009); Use of FRNA bacteriophages to indicate the risk of norovirus contamination in Irish Oysters; *Journal of Family Practice* 72(11):2358–2362

Formiga-Cruz, M., A.K. Allard, A.C. Conden-Hansson, K. Henshilwood, B.E. Hernroth, J. Jofre, D.N. Lees, F. Lucena, M. Papapetropoulou, R.E. Rangdale, A. Tsibouxi, A. Vantarakis and R. Girones (2003); Evaluation of potential indicators of viral contamination in shellfish and their applicability to diverse geographical areas; *Applied and Environmental Microbiology* 69(3):1556–1563

Heras, H., J. Kean-Howie and R.G. Ackman (1994); The potential use of lipid microspheres as nutritional supplements for adult *Ostrea edulis*; *Aquaculture* 123(3–4):309–322

Hernroth, B.E., A-C. Conden-Hansson, A-S. Rehnstam-Holm, R. Girones and A.K. Allard (2002); Environmental factors influencing human viral pathogens and their potential indicator organisms in the Blue Mussel, *Mytilus edulis*: The first Scandinavian report; *Applied and Environmental Microbiology* 68(9):4523–4533

Iglesias, J.I.P., M.B. Urrutia, E. Navarroa, P. Alvarez-Jornaa, X. Larretxea, S. Bougrierb and M. Heralb (1996); Variability of feeding processes in the cockle *Cerastoderma edule* (L.) in response to changes in seston concentration and composition; *Journal of Experimental Marine Biology and Ecology* 197:121–143

Klumpp, D.W., B.L. Bayne and A.J.S. Hawkins (1992); Nutrition of the giant clam *Tridacna gigas* (L.) I. Contribution of filter feeding and photosynthates to respiration and growth; *Journal of Experimental Marine Biology and Ecology* 155(1):105–122

Laing, I., D.N. Lees, D.J. Page and K. Henshilwood (2004); Research on shellfish cultivation: A synopsis of research funded by the Department for Environment, Food and Rural Affairs (DEFRA) between 1990 and 2003; Science Series Technical Report Number 122; pp. 45–52; Centre For Environment, Fisheries and Aquaculture Science

Landry, E., J.M., Vaughn, T.J. Vicale, and R. Mann (1983); Accumulation of sediment-associated viruses in shellfish; *Applied and Environmental Microbiology* 45(1):238–247

La Rosa, G., Y. Proroga, D. De Medici, F. Capuano, M. Iaconelli, S. Della Libera and E. Sufredini (2017); First detection of hepatitis E virus in shellfish and in seawater from production areas in Southern Italy; *Food and Environmental Virology* [published online]; doi:10.1007/s12560–017–9319-z

Lees, D (2000); Viruses and bivalve shellfish; *International Journal of Microbiology* 59:81–116

Morabia, A. and A. Hardy (2005a); Oysters and enteric fever aetiology in 1900 England; *Journal of Epidemiology and Community Health* 59(2):100

Morabia, A. and A. Hardy (2005b); The pioneering use of a questionnaire to investigate a food borne disease outbreak in early 20th century Britain; *Journal of Epidemiology and Community Health* 59(2):94–9

Polo, D., M. Varela and J. Romalde (2015); Detection and quantification of hepatitis A virus and norovirus in Spanish authorised shellfish harvesting areas; *International Journal of Food Microbiology* 193:43–50

Reizopoulou,S., E. Strogyloudi, A. Giannakourou, K. Pagou, I. Hatzianestis, C. Pyrgaki and E. Granéli (2008); Okadaic acid accumulation in macrofilter feeders subjected to natural blooms of *Dinophysis acuminata*; *Harmful Algae* 7(2):228–234

Rippey, S.R. (1994); Infectious diseases associated with molluscan shellfish consumption; *Clinical Microbiology Reviews* 7(4):419–425

Romalde, J.L., E. Area, G. Sánchez, C. Ribeo, I. Torrado, X. Abad, R.M. Pinto, J.L. Barja and A. Bosch (2002); Prevalence of enterovirus and hepatitis A virus in bivalve molluscs from Galicia (NW Spain): Inadequacy of the EU standards of microbiological quality; *International Journal of Food Microbiology* 74:119–130

Schwab, K.J., F.H. Neill, M.K. Estes, T.G. Metcalf and R.L. Atmar (1998); Distribution of Norwalk virus within shellfish following bioaccumulation and subsequent depuration by detection using RT-PCR; *Journal Of Food Protection* 61(12):1674–1680

Shumway, S.E., T.L. Cucci, R.C. Newell and C.M. Yentsch (1985); Particle selection, ingestion, and absorption in filter-feeding bivalves: *Journal of Experimental Marine Biology and Ecology* 91(1–2):77–92

Sidari, L., P. Nichetto, S. Cok, S. Sosa, A. Tubaro, G. Honsell and R. Della Loggia (1998); Phytoplankton selection by mussels, and diarrhetic shellfish poisoning; *Marine Biology* 131:103–111

Stirling, H.P. and I. Okumus (1995); Growth and production of mussels *(Mytilus edulis* L.) suspended at salmon cages and shellfish farms in two Scottish sea lochs; *Aquaculture* 134:93–210

Straub, T.M., K.H. zu Bentrup, P. Orosz-Coghlan, A. Dohnalkova, B.K. Mayer, R.A. Bartholomew, C.O. Valdez, C.J. Bruckner-Lea, C.P. Gerba, M. Abbaszadegan, and C.A. Nickerson (2007); In vitro cell culture infectivity assay for human noroviruses; *Emerging Infectious Diseases* 13(3):396–403

Suzuki, T. and T. Mitsuya (2001); Comparison of dinophysistoxin-1 and esterified dinophysistoxin-1 (dinophysistoxin-3) contents in the scallop *Patinopecten yessoensis* and the mussel *Mytilus galloprovincialis*, *Toxicon* 39:905–908.

Tian, P., A. Engelbrektson, X. Jan, W. Zhong and R. Mandrell (2007); Norovirus recognizes histo-blood group antigens on gastrointestinal cells of clams, mussels and oysters: A possible mechanism of bioaccumulation; *Journal of Food Protection* 70(9):2140–2147

3 Smoked fishery products

Smoking was a traditional process used to preserve fish before canning or freezing was available. Fish can be hot or cold smoked, according to the temperature of the smoke. Hot smoked fish are usually processed so that the internal temperature of the fish exceeds 60°C (Busta *et al.* 2001). This provides a cooking stage in the process. Cold smoked fish is rarely heated to temperatures above 38°C, so it is effectively still a raw product. The hazards associated with smoked products will differ according to whether they are cold or hot smoked.

Smoking process

Smoking (hot or cold) is multi-stage. Preservation is the result of a hurdle process, using several measures to control bacterial growth. The process is summarised in Table 3.1.

Preparation

Nearly all fish are eviscerated prior to smoking. Bloaters are the one type of smoked product where the guts are left intact. All others are gutted. As mentioned in Chapter 1 on fish parasites, early evisceration is an important control measure to prevent migration of nematode parasites such as *Anisakis simplex* from the gut to the flesh. Fish can be split along the belly or along the backbone, beheaded, boned, skinned or just eviscerated according to the species and product to be made. Table 3.2 lists the common smoked fishery products and their associated processing.

Salting/brining

Salting occurs when the fish is packed into dry salt. Brining is the term used when the fish is immersed in or injected with a salt solution. The step is designed to lower the a_w of the product and act as a barrier to microbial growth. Fish that are salted are usually packed in salt and left at cool temperatures. The length of time needed depends on the size and quality of the fish as well as the ambient temperature. Salting usually takes 12–24 hours but in heavily processed products (e.g. red herrings) can take longer. The salt dissolves in the

Table 3.1 Smoked fish process steps

Step	
Preparation	Cleaning, eviscerating, filleting
Salting or brining	Reduces the a_w
	Product may be dry salted, immersed in brine or brine injected
Drain/rinse and rack	Fish may be hooked individually, or threaded on strings or poles, or laid on racks
Drying	Low temperature with air movement to develop a tacky surface
Smoking (Cold)	Cold smoking is usually less than 40^0C so product is technically 'raw'
Smoking (Hot)	Hot smoking ($50–80^0C$) cooks the product
Cooling	Smoked salmon may be frozen for slicing
Packaging	Products may be open packed or vacuum/MAP packed
Storage/distribution	Temperature control needed especially for low O_2 packaging

Table 3.2 Smoked products

Products	Comments	Hot or cold smoked
Kippers	Herrings split down the back with head, guts and backbone removed. May be dyed or undyed	cold
Kipper fillets	Herring but split down the stomach in the normal way a fish is gutted. Usually dyed	cold
Bloater	Whole cold smoked herring. Guts and roe left in, salted rather than brined. Usually left in dry salt at least overnight. Light smoking	cold
Buckling	Herring beheaded and gutted but leaving any roe in place, brined and hot smoked	hot
Finnian haddock	Haddock gutted in the normal way with the head removed but the backbone left in place. Typically undyed	cold
Arbroath smokies	Haddock, beheaded and gutted, but tied together in pairs by the tail before brining and hot smoking	hot
Golden cutlets	Usually whiting, generally small and poorer quality fish used for golden cutlets. Block fillets dyed a virulent yellow	cold
Smoked white fish fillets	Cod, haddock and whiting are all commonly smoked as fillets. They are brined prior to smoking and may be dyed or undyed. Cod and whiting often have the skin removed, but the skin is kept on the haddock as the flesh is more delicate	cold
Smoked salmon	Gutted, beheaded and filleted in the normal way. Usually dry salted, and may have other ingredients such as brown sugar added. Cold smoked, but unusually it is not cooked prior to eating	cold
Smoked trout	Gutted, beheaded and filleted, brined before smoking	hot
Smoked mackerel	Filleted, brined and either hot or cold smoked. The hot smoked fillets may have peppers or other additions put on the surface post smoking. The hot smoked tend to have a wrinkled skin and denatured flesh	both
Smoked eel	Cleaned and dry salted or brined, hot smoked	hot
Red herring	Gutted and salted for several days, air dried and smoked for several weeks. Very low a_w	cold

water phase of the fish flesh, reducing the a_w and erecting a hurdle for germination and growth of microbes.

Brining has a similar effect, but the fish is immersed in a solution of salt and water (brine) and left to soak. This soaking process is generally shorter than for dry salting – possibly as short as twenty minutes depending on the product and brine strength, but for large fish will obviously be longer. Brining or salting begins the preservation process by reducing the water content of the product and thereby reducing the microbiological loading (Porsby *et al.* 2008). The brining process also helps to develop a surface gloss during the smoking and enhances the taste of the final product. When brining, it is critical to ensure the brine is of the correct strength to provide the needed saltiness in the fish. The brines are usually 60–80% salinity, according to the fish and processing method. Brine strength can be determined using a salinometer. Salinometers float at a given level in brine solutions and will indicate the salt content. However, this is dependent on temperature. Therefore, the temperature of the brine must also be taken to ensure it is correct for the salinometer reading. Traditionally an egg or potato was floated in the liquid to indicate whether the brine had reached the correct salt concentration, but the modern approach to hazard control is to take and record a scientific measurement. The brine may be injected into the product but of course this also adds water, which will increase the drying time at the next step. Colours may be added to the brine to enhance the final appearance of the fish. The brine may be re-used, in which case it needs to be monitored as the drip water from previous batches will dilute it. As the concentration of the salt is diluted, microbiological populations washed off the product will be able to survive and multiply, causing a contamination problem for subsequent batches.

Drying

After salting or brining, the fish is dried. This can be done in chill rooms or, traditionally, by wind and sun. Kilic (2009) suggests the optimum conditions are low temperature and high air velocity. He recommends 4°C in air speed of 7 m/sec with relative humidity 40–50%. Small smokers can use electric fans to enhance the air movement. The aim is to give surface tackiness to the fillet so that the smoke products can deposit and adhere. The drying process need only last a short time – up to a few hours depending on the conditions. Too long at this stage results in surface drying which prevents the smoke affecting the flesh.

Smoking

Smoking involves suspending the fish above a smoke source. The smoke is usually generated from sawdust or wood chippings, and the species of wood can impart characteristic flavour to the fish. The burning of the fuel needs to be controlled to provide smoke rather than roaring flames, so the ventilation of the container and moisture content of the fuel are important. Phenols and formaldehyde in the smoke convert the brine-solubilised proteins on the surface of the fillet into a smooth, slightly rubbery pellicle. This pellicle acts as a barrier to microrganisms, helping to preserve the food. The chemicals themselves may also be anti-microbial and phenols help prevent fat oxidation. Other constituents in the smoke such as tars, aldehydes and ketones are deposited on the fillet surface, contributing to the characteristic taste and possibly to the keeping qualities of the fish. The fillets need to be arranged so that the smoke reaches the entire surface. Overcrowding or overlapping of fillets will result in some parts not receiving sufficient smoke or a high enough temperature. These parts will then decompose more quickly, and the fillet will become unfit for human consumption.

Cold smoking

Cold smoking is a process where the temperature of the product generally does not reach above 30°C, and certainly not above 40°C. A cold smoked product is still raw. Many are cooked before eating, for example, smoked haddock, but others such as smoked salmon are actually eaten as they are and are classed as ready to eat. As mentioned in Chapter 1, the cold smoking process alone is insufficient to destroy any parasite larvae in the fish.

Hot smoking

Hot smoked products are those where the smoke reaches higher temperatures and cooks the product as well as smoking it. Hot smoked products are ready-to-eat. Hot smoking usually involves temperatures of 50–80°C. This will destroy most non-spore forming organisms provided the fish is maintained at the temperature for sufficient time. The temperature of the smoke also helps to stop enzymatic activity, so natural hydrolytic and other catabolic activities are halted. The time needed to smoke products depends to some extent on their size, but is usually in the region of several hours, although in some instances it can be 12 hours or more.

Post smoking

As with any foodstuff, cooling needs to be as quick as possible. Any surviving organisms or spores may be able to utilise this step for growth if the a_w is high enough. Smoked fish products can be open packed or vacuum/MAP packed. Heavily salted and dried products such as red herrings can be safely stored at ambient temperature, but nearly all other smoked products must be refrigerated or frozen. This is especially important for those in vacuum or MAP packages where *Clostridium botulinum* may flourish.

Hazards

Any smoked products that are ready to eat will be at risk from cross contamination in the same way as any other ready-to-eat products. The lower a_w can provide a small barrier to growth of mesophilic enteric pathogens but is unlikely to be low enough to inhibit them completely. *Staphylococcus aureus* is reported as halotolerant, growing down to an a_w of 0.86 (Jay 1996), so it will be able to grow and produce toxins in open packed product if cross contamination from handlers occurs post processing.

The main hazards associated with smoked products, particularly vacuum and MAP packed smoked products are *Clostridium botulinum, Listeria monocytogenes*, parasites and possibly histamine development.

Clostridium botulinum

Clostridium botulinum type E is a major concern for smoked fish products. The organism is widespread in aquatic environments and has been isolated from a variety of fish species (Gram 2001b). The organism is spore forming, and neither cold nor hot smoking will reach temperature high enough to inactivate the spores. Gram (2001b) suggests that the hot smoking could actually act as an activation step for spores, thereby increasing the risk. *Clostridium botulinum* is an obligate anaerobe, and the vacuum and MAP packaging methods favoured by smoked fish manufacturers provide ideal conditions for growth. However, there are some reports in the literature of toxin formation in air packaged product (see Gram 2001b) – presumably anaerobic pockets or areas of negative Eh can occur in the product whatever the packaging. Perhaps unsurprisingly, given the temperature of the oceans in which it is found (North Atlantic and North Pacific) *Clostridium botulinum* type E is psychrotrophic. Using temperature as a single control measure to restrict growth is probably only feasible if the product is frozen. An a_w below 0.97 is required to inhibit growth (Jay 1996), and the salting and drying stages assist in reducing the a_w. However, the organism is less tolerant of salt (i.e. more inhibited) as the temperature reduces, so generally the inhibition of this organism is achieved by using a hurdle effect combining a high salt content (lowered a_w) with chill temperatures. According to the ACMSF (1992), fish with 3.5% NaCl (water phase throughout the product) will have a safe storage period of ten days if stored below $10^{0}C$. Temperature control throughout the chain is absolutely essential, especially for fish packed in low O_2 packaging. The Food Standards Agency (2017) guidelines on the safety and shelf-life of vacuum and modified atmosphere packed chilled foods give valuable advice which is relevant to smoked fish products.

Listeria monocytogenes

Listeria monocytogenes is considered a hazard for cold smoked ready-to-eat products such as smoked salmon because it is a psychrotrophic, halotolerant organism and a common environmental contaminant. High risk groups such as pregnant women, immunocompromised individuals, the young and elderly are at particular risk from this organism, and in these groups the mortality rate can be high (Gram 2001a). Innoculation studies using cold smoked salmon (Porsby *et al.* 2008) show that the hurdles of salting, drying and smoking will reduce the bacterial loading of *Listeria monocytogenes*. However, these steps did not eliminate it. Gram (2001a) cites many studies that report growth of *Listeria monocytogenes* in smoked fish products, so it is essential that the requirements of EC Regulation 2073/2005 for *Listeria* in ready-to-eat foods be adhered to and good temperature control be maintained throughout the chain. Recent sampling of smoked products in Italy found that approximately 20% tested positive for *Listeria*, with a small number (3%) failing to meet the <100cfu/g criteria set by Regulation (EC) 2073/2005. Although the sampling was carried out in Italy, the products were manufactured in 12 different EU countries and the level of contamination varied significantly between manufacturers. Some consistently produced contaminated products while others did not. The researchers also found that samples from the same manufacturer tested positive for a particular type of *Listeria*, supporting the idea that *Listeria* will persist in a food business once it has been introduced (Acciari *et al.* 2017). The control of *Listeria* in manufacturers is essential and the Scotland Food Standards Agency (n/d) has produced an online tool which identifies the impact of the steps in the smoking process on *Listeria* contamination. Each step is evaluated through question and answer; the result is supported by clear explanation and then linked to the scientific research papers that provide evidence for the judgement.

Parasites

The parasites associated with eating raw or under processed fish are discussed in Chapter 1 on fish parasites. Cold smoked products that are eaten raw (e.g. smoked salmon) are the highest risk. Products that are cooked before consumption are the lowest risk. Smoked salmon often incorporates a freeze stage after smoking to allow for thin slicing. However, this short freeze may be insufficient to render the product safe and most guidance recommends the product be frozen before processing begins. Farmed salmon are considered to be a much lower risk than wild caught. This is because most are fed pelletised feed which will be free from larval stages. Surveys reported by Beldsoe and Oria (2001) indicate that farmed fish are generally free from anisakid larvae.

Scombrotoxin formation (histamine)

Hot smoking is likely to inhibit the bacteria responsible for histamine production, so provided the fish is kept chilled (on ice) or frozen prior to processing, and the brining and drying processes are also carried out at low temperatures, the production of scombrotoxin should be reasonably well controlled. Theoretically, cold smoking would not destroy the bacteria involved and the elevated temperature during the smoking process could enhance histamine production. However, this theoretical risk does not seem to be reflected in the sampling or food poisoning data. There is only one report in the literature of a smoked product testing positive for histamine and this at relatively low levels (Auerswald *et al.* 2006).

Researchers suggest that cold smoked products do not appear to constitute a high risk for scombrotoxin poisoning but are unable to explain why (Flick *et al.* 2001).

HACCP

One of the difficulties in producing a HACCP plan with repeatable control measures for smoked fishery products is that there is considerable variability in the raw material. A species will differ in fat content, for example, according to whether it is about to spawn or has just finished. The microflora and parasitism will differ according to the geography, and the size and quality of the flesh also varies according to the catch. This means that it could be difficult to set specific parameters that will apply to every fish fillet in the premises. Farmed fish can help standardise the process but not all species are farmed. Another difficulty is that the actual control measures (e.g. the a_w or salt content of the fish or the quantity of antimicrobials deposited during the smoking process) are difficult to measure directly. Salt content, for example must be inferred from measurements of brine salinity and time. Time required in the smoke can be measured as can the internal temperature of the fish, but because of the inherent variability in the raw product this is difficult to standardise.

References

Acciari, V., M. Torresi, L. Iannetti, S. Scattolini, F. Pomilio, L. Decastelli, S. Colmegna, R. Muliari, T. Bossu, Y. Proroga, C. Montagna, C. Cardamone, P. Cogoni, V. Prencipe and G. Migliorati (2017); *Listeria monocytogenes* in smoked salmon and other smoked fish at retail in Italy: Frequency of contamination and strain characterization in products from different manufacturers; *Journal of Food Protection* 80(2):271–278

ACMSF (1992); Report on Vacuum Packaging and Associated Processes; HMSO

Auerswald, L., C. Morren and A. Lopata (2006); Histamine levels in seventeen species of fresh and processed South African seafood; *Food Chemistry* 98:231–239

Beldsoe, G. and M. Oria (2001); Potential hazards in cold-smoked fish: parasites; *Journal of Food Science* 66S(7):S1100–S1103

Busta, F., G.E. Flick, L. Gram, D. Herman, M.L. Jahncke and D. Ward (2001); Processing parameters needed to control pathogens in cold smoked fish; *Journal of Food Science* 66S(7):S1055–S1066

Flick, G., M. Oria and L. Douglas (2001); Potential hazards in cold-smoked fish: Biogenic Amines; *Journal of Food Science* 66S(7):S1088–S1099

Food Standards Agency (2017); The safety and shelf-life of vacuum and modified atmosphere packed chilled foods with respect to non-proteolytic *Clostridium botulinum;* https://www.food.gov.uk/sites/default/files/multimedia/pdfs/publication/vacpacguide. pdf accessed November 2017

Food Standards Agency (Scotland) (n/d); Safe smoked fish assessment; http://safesmokedfish. foodstandards.gov.scot/name-your-assessment/5121 accessed November 2017

Gram, L. (2001a); Potential hazards in cold-smoked fish: *Listeria monocytogenes*; *Journal of Food Science* 66S(7):S1072–S1081

Gram, L. (2001b); Potential hazards in cold-smoked fish: *Clostridium botulinum* Type E; *Journal of Food Science* 66S(7):S1082–S1087

Jay, J. (1996); *Modern Food Microbiology*; 5th edition, Springer

Kilic, A. (2009); Low temperature and high velocity (LTHV) application in drying: Characteristics and effects on the fish quality; *Journal of Food Engineering* 91(1):173–182

Porsby, C., B. Vogel, M. Mohr and L. Gram (2008); Influence of processing steps in cold-smoked salmon production on survival and growth of persistent and presumed non-persistent *Listeria monocytogenes*; *International Journal of Food Microbiology* 122(2008):287–295

4 Outbreaks associated with fruit and vegetables

Meat, poultry, dairy and other high protein foods are traditionally identified as foods that can support pathogenic growth and therefore cause food poisoning. This is still true, and there have been a number of high profile outbreaks involving such foods (e.g. Cowden *et al.* 2001, Pennington 2009). However there have also been a number of well-documented outbreaks in various countries where fruit and vegetables have been implicated as the causative foodstuff. Between 1992 and 2000, 5.5% (83) of the 1,518 foodborne outbreaks of Infectious Intestinal Disease (IID) in England and Wales were associated with the consumption of salad vegetables or fruit (Long *et al.* 2002). A significant number of people were affected (3,438), and there were a total of 69 hospital admissions and one death. Fruit and vegetables have also been identified as causing significant morbidity and mortality in North America, and the contribution appears to be increasing. Sivapalasingam *et al.* (2004) report that fruit and vegetables were implicated in 0.7% of reported foodborne outbreaks in the US in the 1970s, rising to 6% of outbreaks in the 1990s. Fruit and vegetable related outbreaks continue to be reported (Anonymous 2008a). For example, a multistate outbreak of *Listeria* associated with cantaloupe was reported in the USA during the summer/autumn of 2011 (CDC 2011) and an outbreak of *E. coli* O104 associated with sprouted seeds caused significant morbidity and mortality in Europe in the spring and summer of the same year (Frank *et al.* 2011).

Some of the outbreaks are considered to be viral in origin, but those caused by bacterial pathogens commonly involve *Salmonella* or pathogenic *E. coli. Shigella* and *Campylobacter* have also been implicated but the *Salmonella* and pathogenic *E. coli* seem to be particularly well-placed to use fruit and vegetables as carriers. Table 4.1 shows some outbreaks that have been investigated and reported. There appear to be several reasons why *Salmonella* and pathogenic *E. coli* are particularly associated with fruit and vegetable related outbreaks. One is that they are common gut inhabitants of mammals and therefore associated with farmyard manure. Both can survive for long periods in the manure or in water that has been contaminated by animal or human faeces. This provides the route by which contamination of the plants can occur. Vegetables such as lettuce and herbs such as parsley and coriander (cilantro) are eaten raw and have the correct composition

Table 4.1 Outbreaks associated with fruit or vegetables

Outbreak organism	Foodstuff	Country	Reference
Escherichia coli O157:H7	Lettuce	USA	Ackers *et al.* 1998
Salmonella Newport	Salads	UK	Ward *et al.* 2002
Salmonella Typhimurium DT 104	Products containing salads	UK	Anonymous 2000
Escherichia coli O157:H7	Sprouted radish	Japan	Abe *et al.* 2002
Salmonella Kottbus	Sprouted alfalfa	USA	Winthrop *et al.* 2003
Salmonella Poona	Cantaloupe	USA	Anderson *et al.* 2002
Escherichia coli O157:H7	Apple juice	USA	CDC 1996
Salmonella Baildon	Diced tomatoes	USA	Weissinger *et al.* 2000

(pH, a_w, Eh) to support bacterial survival and, in some cases, growth (Islam *et al.* 2004). However, there are other characteristics which make these organisms particularly difficult to control in the context of fruit and vegetable contamination. One issue is their acid tolerance. A second is their ability to attach to surfaces. The third is the potential for internalisation.

Acid

Many fruits are acidic. The US Food and Drug Administration (FDA) website lists strawberries as having a pH of 3.0–3.9, while apple puree and apple juice range from 3.1–3.6 and 3.35–4.0 respectively (FDA 2007). For pathogens such as *S. aureus*, this is too acidic, and they would not survive well (Jay 1996). However, both *Salmonella* and *E. coli* have what is known as an Acid Tolerance Response (ATR). When these organisms are placed in an environment containing organic acids such as acetic or proprionic, the acids can diffuse into the cell. This diffusion causes a decrease in cytoplasmic pH, which acts as a shock to the organism. The shock triggers a response which includes increasing the removal of H+ from the cell (to increase the pH), altering the membrane composition and synthesising protective and repair proteins. These responses help the cell to withstand what would normally be lethal pH conditions of less than 4 (Rodriguez-Romo and Yousef 2006). Growing in mild acid conditions (e.g. pH 5.8) or 'pre-stressing' enhances the resistance and also, unfortunately, appears to provide cross tolerance to other shocks such as heat and salt (Bearson *et al.* 1998). Under experimental conditions Yu *et al.* (2001) report *E. coli* O157 survived for three days in strawberries with a pH 3.5–3.7 and longer in pulps (four days at pH 2.51 or 30 days at pH 3.1). Marques *et al.* (2001) inoculated *E. coli* O157 into fruit pulps and also found lengthy survival – up to 30 days in pH ranges 3.24–2.78 at 4°C. Sharma *et al.* (2001) report survival of *Salmonella* for 32 days in orange juice, pH 3.9. The inoculated organisms did not appear to grow under these conditions but did survive satisfactorily. For an organism such as *E. coli* O157 with a small infectious dose, survival is likely to be sufficient to cause an outbreak. It is possible that the low temperatures at which these experiments were conducted had an effect on the growth rate as shown by Weissinger *et al.* (2000), who isolated *Salmonella* baildon from an infected patient and inoculated the organism onto cut tomatoes. They were able to show a 4 log increase in 24 hours at 21°C. Ukuku and Sapers (2001) were also able to show growth when inoculated cantaloupe (*Salmonella* Stanley) was stored above 4°C. Certainly, various *Salmonella* serovars have been implicated in fruit and vegetable outbreaks, indicating that an infectious dose is potentially achievable in normal food preparation situations.

Attachment

There are a number of plant-associated bacteria whose attachment mechanisms have been studied. These include symbionts such as the *Rhizobium* species that fix nitrogen in legumes, as well as plant pathogens and spoilage organisms such as *Erwinia* and *Pseudomonas.* Such microbes use a variety of attachment mechanisms to adhere to the plants. These include the use of fimbriae, pili and flagella as well as the secretion of specific molecules with specificity for receptor sites on the plant. An example of the latter would be the secretion of the protein RS–IIL which has a specificity for the fruit sugar D-fructose, resulting in an adhesion (Mandrell *et al.* 2006). Some of these proteins are common to both the plant-associated microbes and to those associated with the mammalian gut such as *E. coli*. Some of the gram-negative bacteria that act as plant pathogens and spoilage organisms use what is known as a Type III secretion system to adhere to the plant cells. Both *Salmonella* and *E. coli* (also gram negative) use a Type III secretion system to adhere to the intestinal cells of their mammalian hosts (Mandrell *et al.* 2006). It would appear that these attachment systems used by *Salmonella* and *E. coli* work well in human intestines and also in plant material (Frankel 2008). The significance of these attachment mechanisms is that they form a chemical bond between the organism and the plant. This bond is not one that can be easily disrupted by washing, even in chlorinated water.

Research carried out on the place of attachment shows that organisms favour certain attachment sites such as stem scars, damaged areas and cut surfaces (Takeuchi *et al.* 2001, Wachtel and Charkowski 2002). Iturriaga *et al.* (2007) inoculated tomatoes with an outbreak strain of *S.* Montevideo and found survival under all incubation conditions, growth under most and biofilm formation in some circumstances.

Attachment appears to occur quickly on cut surfaces (Mandrell *et al.* 2006,) and the organisms attached to cut surfaces cannot usually be removed by normal washing methods (Weissinger *et al.* 2000). Cutting through contaminated surfaces can actually transfer the organisms to the flesh of a fruit (Ukuku and Sapers (2001) where growth can occur if conditions are propitious. The acid tolerance response mentioned previously also appears to be enhanced when the organism is attached to a cut surface (Gawande and Bhagwat 2002).

Internalisation

Under certain circumstances it would appear that bacteria can become internalised into plants, meaning they are located within the plant tissue. Bacteria can enter the plant through natural openings such as the stomata or through damaged areas and wounds. One specialised place where wound formation is likely to offer opportunity for human pathogen internalisation is during root growth. The emergence of a root tip causes a wound in the plant tissue which allows colonisation by soil bacteria. The use of contaminated irrigation water or manure could provide a source of organisms such as *Salmonella* and *E. coli* which could enter the plant during root growth. Experimental work has shown that *E. coli* O157 can enter the seedlings of cabbage and lettuce and remain in the plant tissue until maturity (Wachtel *et al.* 2002a and 2002b; Solomon *et al.* 2002). Shi *et al.* (2007) inoculated *Salmonella* onto tomato flowers and tested the fruit that developed. The researchers found internalised and externalised persistence of the serovars in the fruit. Although Miles *et al.* (2009) did not identify internalisation from irrigation water under experimental conditions, it is possible that contaminated water falling on the growing sections of the plant could act as a source for internalised bacteria, particularly if aerosolised (Bartz 2006). Sprinkler irrigation systems can disperse aerosols very long distances.

Once harvested, produce is still at risk from internalisation of bacteria. As fresh produce cools, the internal pressure can be reduced. If this takes place while the product is submerged in water, it will tend to absorb water to try and equilibrate. Water will be absorbed through any damaged or cut areas and also through blossom scars. Bartz (2006) reports various researchers as having shown not just uptake of water and dye, but also internalisation of pathogens through this process. Apples submerged in water contaminated with *E. coli* and mangos in a suspension of *Salmonella* both internalised the pathogens during the cooling process. Apparently, pressure washing and the use of heavy jets of water could have the same effect (Bartz 2006).

Outbreaks

Table 4.1 gives examples of outbreaks that are considered to have been caused by contaminated fruit or vegetables. There are some characteristics that are common to these outbreaks. Because the contamination incident often occurs on the farm or at the processor, the number of cases can be substantial and may be spread over a large geographic area. For example, there were three outbreaks identified in the US in 2000, 2001 and 2002 involving cantaloupe and *Salmonella* Poona. These were multi-state outbreaks, and the 2002 incident involved Canada as well. The whole cantaloupes came from farms in Mexico, and the 2001 and 2002 Pulsed

Field Gel Electrophoresis (PFGE) patterns were indistinguishable, suggesting a common persistent contamination source. In total there were 155 laboratory confirmed cases (Anderson *et al.* 2002). An outbreak in the US in 1996 caused by *E. coli* O157:H7 on mesclun lettuce was multi-state also, with at least 61 patients, three of whom developed Haemolytic Uremic Syndrome (HUS) (Ackers *et al.* 1998). A more recent outbreak associated with peppers (and possibly tomato) caused illness in 1,442 patients across 43 states in the US, plus Washington, DC, and Canada in 2008 (Anonymous 2008a).

Another common characteristic of fruit and vegetable outbreaks is a complex distribution chain. Packers or processors frequently use the product of more than one farm in a batch, and any one packer or processor may supply to a number of wholesalers. These wholesalers can use more than one supplier for the same product which will complicate the investigation.

Because the contamination incident often occurs early in the food chain, inspections of the retailer or restaurant supplying the food may not provide any useful information.[1] In some outbreaks there will also be cases that have handled the food at home perfectly correctly but still have still been affected (Weissinger *et al.* 2000; Anderson *et al.* 2002).

During the investigation it can also be difficult to get accurate food histories because salad vegetables are often used as a garnish. People report eating meat products or other foods without remembering that there was a salad or herb garnish. Even when prompted, patients may not be able to recall accurately. This makes identifying a food association and calculating any statistics more difficult. It is important to ask the chef for details of how the meals are plated to ensure garnishes, final sprinkles of herbs and decorations are included in the investigation.

Summary

The characteristics of the pathogens described in this chapter make certain organisms likely to be associated with fruit and vegetable products. In addition, some of the production methods (irrigation, washing, chopping, waxing) appear to enhance the likelihood that the pathogens will survive in such a way that they cannot be removed before ingestion. The Food Standards Agency and other organisations are encouraging people to increase their consumption of fruit and vegetables to ensure a healthy diet. As the consumption of a food stuff increases, the associated morbidity also usually increases. This is likely to be the case with fruit and vegetable related outbreaks, especially because in many production areas there is intense pressure on water, making the use of potable water for irrigation and processing less and less likely (Anonymous 2008b).

Note

1 Of course it is perfectly possible for a restaurant to contaminate a batch of sliced tomatoes in the kitchen and poison its customers. In such a situation, the distribution of cases will resemble a normal point source outbreak rather than the widespread distribution described previously.

References

Anonymous (2000); Case control study links salad vegetables to national increase in multi-resistant *Salmonella* Typhimurium DT 104; *CDR Weekly* 10(37):333–336

Anonymous (2008a); Investigation of Outbreak of Infections Caused by *Salmonella* Saintpaul; http://www.cdc.gov/Salmonella/saintpaul/

Anonymous (2008b); Rethinking California's Irrigation Strategy; http://www.planetizen.com/node/34413

Abe, K., S. Yamamoto, and K. Shinagawa (2002); Economic impact of an *Escherichia coli* O157:H7 outbreak in Japan; *Journal of Food Protection* 65(1):66–72

Ackers, M.L., B.E. Mahon, E. Leahy, B. Goode, T. Damrow, P.S. Haynes, W.F. Bibb, D.H. Rice, T.J. Barrett, L. Hutwagner, P.M. Griffin and L. Slutsker (1998); An outbreak of *Escherichia coli* O157:H7 Infections associated with leaf lettuce consumption; *Journal of Infectious Diseases* 177:1588–93

Anderson, S.M., L. Verchick, M.S. Clarke, R. Sowadsky, R. Civen, J.C. Mohle-Boetani, S.B. Werner, M. Starr, S. Abbott, M. Gutierrez, M. Palumbo, J. Farrar, P. Shillam, E. Umland, M. Tanuz, M. Sewell, J. Cato, W. Keene, M. Goldoft, J. Hoffman, J. Kobayashi, P. Waller, C. Braden, M. Reler and W. Chege (2002); Multistate outbreaks of *Salmonella* serotype Poona infections associated with eating cantaloupe from Mexico-United States and Canada, 2000–2002; *Journal of the American Medical Association* 288(23):2967–2969

Bartz, J. (2006) Internalization and infiltration; In *Microbiology of Fruits and Vegetables,* eds. G. Sapers, J. Gorny, A. Yousef; pp. 75–94; Taylor and Francis; New York

Bearson, B.L., L. Wilson and J. Foster (1998); A low pH –inductible PhoPQ-dependent acid tolerance response protects *Salmonella* Typhimurium against inorganic acid stress; *Journal of Bacteriology* 180(9):2409–2417

Centers for Disease Control and Prevention (CDC) (1996); Outbreak of *Escherichia coli* O157:H7 infections associated with drinking unpasteurized commercial apple juice – British Columbia, California, Colorado and Washington October 1996; http://www.cdc.gov.epo/mmwr/preview/mmwrhtml/00044358.htm

Centers for Disease Control and Prevention (CDC) (2011); Multistate outbreak of Listeriosis linked to whole cantaloupes from Jensen Farms, Colorado; http://www.cdc.gov/listeria/outbreaks/index.html accessed October 4, 2011

Cowden, J.M., S. Ahmend, M. Donaghy and A. Riley (2001); Epidemiological investigation of the Central Scotland outbreak of *Escherichia coli* O157:H7 infection, November to December 1996; *Epidemiology & Infection* 126: 335–341

FDA (2007); Acidified and low acid canned foods; Approximate pH of Foods and Food Products; http://ucfoodsafety.ucdavis.edu/files/266402.pdf accessed March 15, 2018

Frank, C., D. Werber, J.P. Cramer, M. Askar, M. Faber, M. an der Heiden, H. Bernard, A. Fruth, R. Prager, A. Spode, M. Wadl, A. Zoufaly, S. Jordan, K. Stark, and G. Krause (2011); Epidemic Profile of Shiga-Toxin producing *Escherichia coli* O104:H4 Outbreak in Germany; *New England Journal of Medicine* 365(19):1771–80

Frankel, G. (2008); Attachment of *Escherichia coli* O157:H7 and *Salmonella enteric* to Salad Leaves; Programme and abstracts of 21st ICFMH Symposium, Aberdeen, plenary session 11, p 67

Gawande, P.V. and A.A. Bhagwat (2002); Protective effects of cold temperature and surface-contact on acid tolerance of *Salmonella* spp.; *Journal of Applied Microbiology* 93:689–696

Islam, M; J. Morgan, M.P. Doyle; S.C. Phatak, P. Millner and X. Jiang (2004); Persistence of *Salmonella enterica* serovar Typhimurium on lettuce and parsley and in soils on which they were grown in fields treated with contaminated manure composts or irrigation water; *Foodborne Pathogens and Disease* 1(1):27–35

Jay, J.M. (1996); *Food Microbiology*, 5th edition; Chapman Hill

Iturriaga, M.H., M.L. Tamplin and E.F. Escartin (2007); Colonization of tomatoes by *Salmonella* Montevideo is affected by relative humidity and storage temperature; *Journal of Food Protection* 70(1):30–4

Long, S.M., G.K. Adak, S.J. O'Brien and I.A. Gillespie (2002); General outbreaks of infectious intestinal disease linked with salad vegetables and fruit; *Communicable Disease and Public Health* 5(2):101–5

Mandrell, R., L. Gorski and M. Brandl (2006); Attachment of microorganisms to fresh produce; In: *Microbiology of Fruits and Vegetables*, eds. G. Sapers, J. Gorny, A. Yousef; pp. 33–61; Taylor and Francis; New York

Marques, P.A.H.F., D. Worcman-Barninka, S.C.S. Lannes and M. Landgraf (2001); Acid tolerance and survival of *Escherichia coli* O157:H7 inoculated in fruit pulps stored under refrigeration; *Journal of Food Protection* 64(11):1674–1678

Miles J.S., S.S. Sumner, R.R. Boyer, R.C. Williams, J.G. Latimer and J.G. McKinney (2009) Internalization of *Salmonella enterica* serovar Montevideo into greenhouse tomato plants through contaminated irrigation water or seed stock. *Journal of Food Protection* 72(4):849–52

Pennington, H. (2009); The Public Inquiry into the September 2005 Outbreak of *E. coli* O157 in South Wales; HMSO; http://wales.gov.uk/ecolidocs/3008707/reporten.pdf?skip=1andlang=en accessed June 24, 2011

Rodriguez-Romo, L. and A. Yousef (2006); Microbial stress adaptation and safety of produce; In: *Microbiology of Fruits and Vegetables*, eds. G. Sapers, J. Gorny, A. Yousef; pp. 95–114; Taylor and Francis; New York

Sivapalasingam, S., C. Friedman, L. Cohen and R. Tauxe (2004); Fresh produce: A growing cause of outbreaks of foodborne illness in the United States, 1973 through 1997; *Journal of Food Protection* 67(10):342–2353

Sharma, M., L.R. Beuchat, M.P. Doyle and J. Chen (2001); Survival of *Salmonellae* in pasteurized, refrigerated calcium-fortified orange juice; *Journal of Food Protection* 64(9):1299–1304

Shi, X., A. Namvar, M. Kostrzynska, R. Hora and K. Warriner (2007); Persistence and growth of different *Salmonella* serovars on pre- and post-harvest tomatoes; *Journal of Food Protection* 70(12):2725–31.

Solomon, E.B., S. Yara and K.R. Matthews (2002); Transmission of *Escherichia coli* O157:H7 from contaminated manure and irrigation water to lettuce plant tissue and its subsequent internalization; *Applied and Environmental Microbiology* 68(1):397–400

Takeuchi, K., A.N. Hassan and J.F. Frank (2001); Penetration of *Escherichia coli* O157:H7 into lettuce as influenced by modified atmosphere and temperature; *Journal of Food Protection* 64(11):1820–1823

Ukuku, D. and G. Sapers (2001); Effect of sanitizer treatments on *Salmonella* Stanley attached to the surface of cantaloupe and cell transfer to fresh-cut tissues during cutting practices; *Journal of Food Protection* 64(9):1286–91

Ward, L.R., C. Maguire, M.D. Hampton, E. de Pinna, H.R. Smith, C.L. Littlew, I.A. Gillespie, S.J. O'Brien, R.T. Mitchell, C. Sharpe, R.A. Swann, O. Doyle and E.J. Threlfall (2002); Collaborative investigation of an outbreak of *Salmonella enterica* serotype Newport in England and Wales associated with ready-to-eat salad vegetables; *Communicable Disease and Public Health* 5(4):301–304

Watchel, M.R. and A.O. Charkowski (2002); Cross-contamination of lettuce with *Escherichia coli* O157:H7; *Journal of Food Protection* 65(3):465–470

Wachtel, M.R., L.C. Whitehand and R.E. Mandrell (2002a); Association of *Escherichia coli* O157:H7 with preharvest leaf lettuce upon exposure to contaminated irrigation water; *Journal of Food Protection* 65(1):18–25

Wachtel, M.R., L.C. Whitehand and R.E. Mandrell (2002b); Prevalence of *Escherichia coli* associated with a cabbage crop inadvertently irrigated with partially treated sewage waste water; *Journal of Food Protection* 65(3):471–475

Weissinger, W.R., W. Chantarapanont and L.R. Beuchat (2000); Survival and Growth of *Salmonella* Baildon in shredded lettuce and diced tomatoes, and effectiveness of chlorinated water as a sanitizer; *International Journal of Food Microbiology* 62:123–131

Winthrop, K.L., M.S. Palumbo, J.A. Farrar; J.C. Mohle-Boetani, S. Abbott, M.E. Beatty, G. Inami and S.B. Werner (2003); Alfalfa sprouts and *Salmonella* Kottbus infection: A multistate outbreak following inadequate seed disinfection with heat and chlorine; *Journal of Food Protection* 66(1): 13–17

Yu, K., M.C. Newman, D.D. Archbold and T.R. Hamilton-Kemp (2001); Survival of *Escherichia coli* O157:H7 on strawberry fruit and reduction of the pathogen population by chemical agents; *Journal of Food Protection* 64(9):1334–1340

Websites

FDA http://www.cfsan.fda.gov/~comm/lacf-phs.html

5 Mycotoxins

Mycotoxins are substances that are naturally produced by some fungi. The grouping 'mycotoxin' is an artificial category, in that its members are not defined by any coherent chemical or biological similarities, but because they are all hazardous if ingested by humans or animals. It is not entirely clear why fungi produce these substances. Mycotoxins could just be by-products of the fungal metabolism or they might serve a purpose that is beneficial to the fungi. Some researchers suggest mycotoxin production may be related to environmental or stress adaptation. In the laboratory *Aspergillus flavus* can be shown to increase the production of mycotoxins when subjected to stress, for example osmotic, pH or temperature stress (Geisen *et al.* 2017). Oxidative stress in the form of peroxide has also been shown to enhance aflatoxin production (Kolliputi *et al.* 2006). Some of the fungi that produce mycotoxins are plant pathogens, and it has been postulated that the mycotoxins may have a role to play in the infection process. For example, Desjardins *et al.* (1992) reported that, under laboratory conditions, *Fusarium (Gibberella pulicaris)* could not infect parsnip roots when it was unable to produce the mycotoxin tricothecene, although it could still infect potatoes. Other workers suggest that patulin production by *Penicillium expansum* is important when the fungus colonises apples (Sanzani *et al.* 2012). Whatever functions these substances may serve for the fungi producing them, they are all considered to be toxic to mammals, including humans, and as such need to be eliminated from food and feed as far as is possible.

The fungi which produce mycotoxins tend to infect food plants during growth. Some cause diseases in plants, damaging and reducing the usable crop, as well as producing mycotoxins in the pre-harvest stage (Abbas *et al.* 2016). Some of those which infect the plants during growth/ripening can survive into the post-harvest stages where they continue to produce toxins if conditions are favourable. Staple cereals such as wheat, maize and barley are commonly contaminated with mycotoxin producing fungi, as are peanuts, tree nuts, dried fruit and spices. The mycotoxin patulin (produced by *Penicillium expansum*) is associated with apple products, especially juice. Controls for these 'survivors' need to continue throughout the food chain to ensure stored, processed and packaged food are safe for consumption.

Health impact

The health effects of mycotoxins vary according to many parameters, including the type of mycotoxin, the amount ingested and, to some degree, the health and age of the recipient. Most of the information on health effects has been determined through epidemiological studies (during an outbreak or through geographical associations) or through animal feeding studies. This means the effects of mycotoxin ingestion can be difficult to establish as direct cause and effect but the evidence leaves no doubt that exposure should be avoided as much as possible. The health burden of mycotoxin contamination is considered particularly problematic in developing countries where underlying disease or malnutrition can magnify the effects of exposure (Misihairabgwi *et al.* 2017). Contaminated feed can cause detectable diseases in animals, and in some cases the toxins can persist in the meat, milk or eggs.

Mycotoxins are considered to have potential for both acute and chronic effects. Reports where populations of humans or farm animals have ingested high doses of a mycotoxin in a short time period provide information about acute effects. For example, studies have identified serious kidney disease (nephropathy) in pigs which have eaten feed contaminated with Ochratoxin A (Elling and Moller 1973, Stoev 2013). Fatal liver damage has occurred in poultry which have been fed aflatoxin contaminated feed (Pitt and Miller 2017). Poor growth and changes in blood composition have been demonstrated in chickens exposed to feed contaminated with Deoxynivalenol (DON) and Zearalenone (Swamy *et al.* (2004). Epidemiological evidence suggests that Fumonisin B1 can cause neural tube defects in experimental embryos if the mother ingests contaminated product at critical stages in pregnancy (Stoev 2013). Incidents of humans affected by ingesting highly contaminated food are, fortunately, not common but a serious outbreak of human aflatoxicosis occurred in Kenya in 2004 (Azziz-Baumgartner *et al.* 2005). This outbreak was caused by eating contaminated maize and affected 317 people. They developed acute hepatic failure and 125 died. Sampling of the maize in case households gave an average total aflatoxin level of 354 parts per billion (ppb) (Lewis *et al.* 2005). Commission Regulation (EC) No 1881/2006 sets a max of 10 µ/kg (ppb) for maize to be processed before human consumption.

Long-term lower dose exposure is also considered harmful. Krogh *et al.* (1977) linked Balkan Endemic Nephropathy with persistent exposure to Ochratoxin A through contaminated food. Over a four-year period significantly more samples of cereal in the endemic areas were contaminated than in the control areas. In addition, the levels of contamination in endemic areas could be very high – as much as ten times the maximum level currently permitted by Commission Regulation (EC) No 1881/2006. Exposure to Ochratoxin A has been shown to be immunosuppressive in pigs (Stoev *et al.* 2000) increasing the susceptibility of the animals to secondary bacterial infection. Whether this might also be the case in humans has not been demonstrated but is not impossible. Recent work indicates that Zearalenone is an endocrine disruptor in animals (Lee and Ryu 2015) and in

Table 5.1 Source and health effects of commonly identified mycotoxins

Mycotoxin	Source fungi	Main food associations	Acute	Chronic	Comments
Aflatoxins Aflatoxin B_1, G_1 and G_2 B_2, G_1 and G_2	*Aspergillus flavus A. parasiticus*	Maize, peanuts, tree nuts, dried fruit	Hepatitis and GI symptoms, Ascites Teratogenic and mutagenic	Hepatocellular carcinoma (Liver cancer) IARC Class 1	Can be excreted in milk as M_1 or M_2
Ochratoxin A	*Aspergillus ochraceus Penicillium verrucosum*	Barley wheat rye oats, coffee cocoa soya beans spices nuts fruit	Nephropathy in pigs chickens, rats Animal studies indicate that it is hepatotoxic, immunosuppressant, teratogenic and carcinogenic (testicular cancer)	Some evidence of carcinogenicity in rats IARC Class 2B Association with Balkan Endemic Nephropathy	Pigs and chickens with nephropathy have also had detectable levels in organs and muscle. Egg yolks have tested positive depending on the level in the feed. Has been identified in human milk reflecting maternal ingestion
Patulin	*Penicillium expansum*	Apples and apple products. Can be found on other fruits			Appears to be denatured by fermentation
Fusarium toxins					
Zearalenone	*Fusarium graminearum, F. culmorum F. crookwellense and other Fusarium species*	Predominantly associated with maize but also reported in wheat, beans, soybeans rice, sorghum	Reproductive disruption in pigs, cattle and sheep at very low levels	Endocrine disruptor	Oestrogen mimic (mycoestrogen)
Fumonisin B_1	*Fusarium verticilliodes*	Predominantly associated with maize but also reported in beans, soybeans rice, sorghum and asparagus	In animals: leukoencephalomalacia, pulmonary oedema, hydrothorax, liver damage,	Link with oesophageal cancer and liver cancer in humans, also possibly neural tube defects in embryo	Has been identified in human milk

Tricothecenes: A family of mycotoxins produced by several species

Mycotoxin	Species	Crops	Effects / Symptoms	IARC / Immune	Notes
			carcinoma (liver and kidney), neural tube defects in embryos In humans: GI symptoms	IARC Class 2B	
T-2 HT-2	Fusarium species	Barley wheat rye maize rice	GI, Neurological and dermatologic effects Cytotoxic (inhibit protein synthesis)	Immunosuppressive	Historic association with Alimentary Toxic Aleukia
Nivalenol Deoxynivalenol (DON)	Fusarium species	Barley wheat rye maize safflower seeds	Farm animals: Gastro-intestinal symptoms at high doses, food refusal and weight loss in lower doses Humans: GI symptoms, headache, fever	Immunosuppression in animal studies	Has been detected in liver and kidneys of food species and in eggs and milk
Citrinin	Penicillium species Aspergillus species Monascus species	Barley wheat rye oats, maize rice	Nephrotoxin in animals, No data available for humans		Appears to act synergistically with Ochratoxin A
Ergot alkaloids	Claviceps purpurea	Rye	Humans: St. Anthony's fire (hallucinations and convulsions,) gangrene Animals: convulsions and gangrene, abortion, ataxia, suppression of lactation, hypersensitivity		

Sources: WHO (1990); ESA (2016); Krogh et al. (1977); Azziz-Baumgartner et al. (2004); Bennet & Klich (2003); Stoev (2013); Stein & Bulboaca (2017); Malir et al. (2013)

humans (Kowalska *et al.* 2016). The International Agency for Research on Cancer (IARC; 2017) has classed Aflatoxin B1 and naturally occurring mixes of aflatoxins as group 1 carcinogens (carcinogenic to humans). Other mycotoxins such as Ochratoxin A and Fumonisin B1 are categorised by IARC as possible human carcinogens (group 2B).

The effect of mycotoxin ingestion can be exacerbated by, or impact on, pre-existing health conditions. For example, in the Kenyan aflatoxicosis outbreak, epidemiologists found that patients with acute hepatic failure were significantly more likely to have hepatitis B antigens than the control group (Azziz-Baumgartner *et al.* 2005). Ross *et al.* (1992) assessed development of liver cancer among men in Shanghai and found that while aflatoxin exposure and hepatitis B each increased the risk of developing the cancer slightly (relative risk of 2 and 5 respectively), combined exposure to aflatoxin and hepatitis B increased the risk of developing liver cancer significantly (relative risk of 60).

Table 5.1 summarises the commonly identified mycotoxins, source fungi and the health effects which have so far been identified or proposed. Note that some fungi produce more than one mycotoxin and some mycotoxins are produced by more than one fungus.

Distribution and exposure

Plant based foods are colonised by fungi during growth and ripening. The success of the fungi (and consequent development of mycotoxins) is related to the host plant and to the growth conditions. Some production areas are considered higher risk than others for particular mycotoxins. For example *A. flavus* inhabits warmer parts of the world (Stein and Bulboaca 2017), and its association with fruit and nuts from places like Iran, Turkey, California and Bolivia reflect that distribution. The optimum temperature for Ochratoxin A production by *P. verrucosum* is 20°C, making it associated with products such as wheat from cooler areas of the world. Of course, Ochratoxin A is also produced by *A. ochreaus* (preferred production temperature 31°C), and so it can contaminate more tropical products such as spices and coffee as well.

The association of mycotoxin producing fungi with so many of the world's basic cereals ensures a wide distribution. Contaminated crops may find their way directly into food production or be used as animal feed. Products of animal origin such as eggs and milk have tested positive for Ochratoxin A, as has pork (Bennet and Klich 2003). Aflatoxins M_1 and M_2 are the metabolised forms of aflatoxins B_1 and B_2 which have been ingested as part of the feed and excreted by the cow in her milk (Stein and Bulboaca 2017). Sampling of food suggests widespread contamination. For example, in the US, sampling of breakfast cereals available at retail identified Ochratoxin A in 42% of them. Oat based cereals were the most frequently contaminated in this survey, with 70% testing positive. The researchers also found contamination in infant oat based cereals at levels which would be prohibited if found on sale in the EU (Lee and Ryu 2015). Similar sampling on breakfast cereals was carried out in 2014 in Lisbon, Portugal by Martins *et al.* (2018).

The study identified the presence of a mycotoxin in 96% of the cereals tested. All were below EU maximum permitted limits according to Commission Regulation (EC) No 1881/2006 but 92% tested positive for more than one mycotoxin. The health implication of simultaneous exposure to low levels of multiple mycotoxins is unknown (Stoev 2013) but some researchers feel it may be extremely significant (Malir *et al.* 2013, Stoev 2013).

Surveillance on humans supports the concept of widespread low-level exposure, although the impact is uncertain. Not all mycotoxin exposure can be easily measured. Ochratoxin A has a long half-life (approximately 35 days) in humans and can be identified through blood samples (Lee and Ryu 2015). Aflatoxin B_1 can be detected in the urine (short term exposure) and also forms lysine adducts which are persistent in the serum. These can be used to measure exposure over longer periods (months). Other mycotoxins are more difficult to evaluate due to the way they are metabolised or to lack of reliable correlation between the products measured and exposure (Lee and Ryu 2015). Reports from the 1990s suggest that one fifth of the people tested in France, 97% of people in Italy (Abouzied *et al.* 2002) and 98% of people tested in Germany (Rosner *et al.* 2000) had detectable levels of Ochratoxin A in their blood. A more recent survey in Italy (di Giuseppe *et al.* 2012) identified Ochratoxin A in 99.1% of the participants, confirming that in this country the levels appear unchanged. The authors suggest wine and coffee as among the important potential sources. Misihairabgwi *et al.* (2017) evaluate the exposure of consumers in the countries of southern Africa. There is concern that exposure in developing countries is more significant for several reasons. Consumers in developing countries may have a less varied diet, relying heavily on single staples such as maize. Mycotoxin contamination in a staple food is likely to have an enhanced impact because an individual will consume proportionally more of it than if a diverse diet is available. Any underlying levels of poor health will exacerbate the effect of the contamination as described previously in the Kenyan aflatoxin outbreak (Azziz-Baumgartner *et al.* 2005) and the Shanghai liver cancer study (Ross *et al.* 1992). Foods for domestic consumption in developing countries are considered more likely to be contaminated with mycotoxins and at higher levels than elsewhere (Misihairabgwi *et al.* 2017; Stoev 2013; Medina *et al.* 2017) because the products with low levels of contamination tend to be exported, as they will be compliant with the maximum levels set by places like the EU. This leaves the non-compliant contaminated foods for consumption in the producing country.

Control

The fungi which produce mycotoxins are endemic in the relevant crop-growing regions and persist in soil so there is always the potential for infection. The extent of contamination may vary from season to season, increasing when climatic conditions favour the growth of invading fungi at the expense of the crop. For example, increased aflatoxin production can be observed on maize and other crops under drought conditions (Bennet and Klich 2003, Medina *et al.* 2017). The first step in controlling mycotoxins is good pre-harvest agricultural practice, in particular irrigation, pest control and good hygiene. A study of aflatoxin levels in four Greek pistachio orchards demonstrated that while aflatoxin could be detected at maturity (when the shell hardens and splits) in all four establishments, the lowest levels were in the orchard which practiced regular irrigation, application of fertiliser and, very importantly, pest control (Georgiadou *et al.* 2012). Sommer *et al.* (1986) working in California pistachio orchards also emphasise the role of insect pests in aflatoxin formation, especially when dealing with early splitter nuts which tend to be at higher risk of infection with *A. flavus*. While approximately 20% of the early splitter nuts without visible insect damage tested positive for aflatoxins, up to 75% of the insect damaged nuts were positive. Dowd (2001) reported that Bt maize which had been genetically modified to be resistant to corn borers also had lower levels of fumonisins compared to the non-Bt maize, simply because there was less physical damage to the corn which helped protect the corn from *Fusarium* colonisation. The total fumonisin levels in the maize correlated with the extent of insect damage. Good Agricultural Practice (GAP) also extends to removing debris and ground litter which can enhance fungal survival and readiness for the next crop (Doster and Michailides (1994).

Post-harvest conditions are also critical in the control of mycotoxins because many can continue to develop during storage. In the Kenyan aflatoxin outbreak it would appear that, owing to food shortages caused by an untimely and inadequate rainy season, many people chose to store the maize in their homes instead of in purpose-built granaries. It was felt to be more secure from theft in the home. Unfortunately the granaries were better ventilated than the homes, allowing the grain to dry and remain dry while the raised storage protected from insects. Although the maize probably had a high contamination rate anyway, due to the drought, sampling revealed that the maize from the households suffering from aflatoxicosis had much higher levels of aflatoxins than the controls (unaffected households). Storage at home was significantly associated with case households suggesting that home storage, with its damp and poorly ventilated conditions was a contributor to the outbreak. Thorough drying and good storage reduce the potential for mycotoxin formation by controlling the growth of any fungi present. It is considered that cereals with less than 15% moisture will not support mycotoxin formation (Stoev 2013, Stein and Bulboaca, 2017), but this could be difficult to achieve and maintain in a domestic environment. In the study of Greek pistachio orchards referred to previously, one orchard with mean aflatoxin contamination slightly above EU standards was able to reduce that to 'not detected' through mechanical drying, sorting and controlled storage at 5–7°C, 45–60% relative humidity. By comparison a second orchard, whose mean contamination at harvest was also somewhat above EU standards, did not follow such good post-harvest processing. The nuts from this orchard were sun-dried and stored at ambient temperature and humidity. Within six weeks, the aflatoxin levels had increased from approximately 34 µ/kg to 371 µ/kg. Commission Regulation (EC) No 1881/2006 sets a maximum of 10 µ/kg total aflatoxin for nuts which are to be sorted or processed and 4 µ/kg for nuts to be used directly for human consumption, meaning these nuts were non-compliant and could not be placed on the market.

Post-harvest protection from pests is also considered important in preventing the development of mycotoxins. The researchers in the Greek pistachio study observed that the highly contaminated nuts were also heavily infested with stored product insects while in the warehouse. A positive correlation between high mycotoxin levels and heavy insect infestation is reported by number of researchers (Sommer *et al.* 1986). Apart from the physical damage caused by the insects which may offer access for the fungi, Udomkun *et al.* (2017) suggest that the respiration from insects will increase the temperature and moisture content of the grains, favouring fungal growth.

Post-harvest sorting can reduce the contamination by the physical removal of contaminated product or the contaminated parts of a product. Sieving and sorting maize to remove obviously damaged and contaminated grains can reduce the contamination levels (Stein and Bulboaca 2017). Stoev (2013) lists a number of examples where researchers report reductions in contamination of various cereals through physical sorting methods. Milling and further processing of cereals may reduce levels in some cases, for example Stein and Bubloaca (2017) report that Ochratoxin A is concentrated in grain husks which are removed during processing. Physical sorting using a variety of techniques (e.g. floating, colour sorting, fluorescence) is part of post-harvest processing for pistachio nuts as well as peanuts (Udomkun *et al.* 2017), and the efficacy of this sorting is reflected in the differing maximum levels given by Commission Regulation (EC) No 1881/2006 according to whether sorting will take place or not. The removal of obviously damaged and rotting apples at all steps is considered critical to minimise patulin during the production of apple juice (OMAFRA 2016). While physical sorting can certainly reduce the level of mycotoxins in a lot or batch of food made of individual units like nuts, there is need for caution. Some officers, food business operators and the public feel that mouldy food (for example hard cheese) can be trimmed and the parts with no visible mould used for human consumption. It should be remembered that the parts of the fungi (the hyphae) which produce the mycotoxins are microscopic and can penetrate into the food without any visible indication. The visible parts – the blue/green/black/white fuzzy material that can be trimmed off easily is actually the reproductive part of the colony (the fruiting bodies) so trimming off what can be seen is unlikely to ensure the removal of hyphae or all the toxins that have been produced. It can only reduce the amount.

Most mycotoxins are heat stable. Ochratoxin A, for example, is stable up to 250°C (Stein and Bulboaca 2017), DON to 350°C (Sobrova *et al.* 2010). This means that, although partial degradation may occur in some processes, normal thermal processing of food and feed is unlikely to render the products completely safe. Table 5.2 summarises some relevant characteristics. Kabak (2008) reviewed the effects of thermal processing on a number of mycotoxins. Although in many cases normal processing methods have been shown to slightly reduce contamination levels, this is variable and dependent on a number of parameters such as substrate, pH, pressure and moisture content. Usually a reduction is observed rather than elimination. In some cases, the treatment needed for elimination is not realistic – for example, the published time: temperature requirements to reduce

Table 5.2 Characteristics of some mycotoxins

Mycotoxin	Source fungi	Degradation temperature	
Aflatoxins Aflatoxin B$_1$ B$_2$, G$_1$ and G$_2$	*Aspergillus flavus* *A. parasiticus*	237–306^{0}C	Partial reductions (30–45%) can be achieved by roasting peanuts at 150^{0}C for 30 minutes. Salt increases the degradation during roasting. Nixtamlization (alkaline cooking) can substantially reduce aflatoxins in tortilla products
Ochratoxin A	*Aspergillus ochraceus* *Penicillum verrucosum*	250^{0}C	
Patulin	*Penicillium expansum*	111^{0}C but acid conditions (pH 3.5–5.5) enhance thermal stability	Fermentation will destroy patulin Optimal patulin production occurs at pH 4 (apple juice is typically 3.5–4)
Fusarium toxins Zearalenone	*Fusarium graminearum,* *F. culmorum* *F. crookwellense* and other *Fusarium* species	Some losses when heated to 150^{0}C for an hour, but >175^{0}C needed (for 1 hour) to reduce >90% (pH 7)	
Fumonisin B$_1$	*Fusarium verticilliodes*		Baking at 200^{0}C reduces by 28% Frying at 190^{0}C reduces by 67%
Tricothecenes T-2 HT-2	*Fusarium* species		
Nivalenol Deoxynivalenol (DON)	*Fusarium* species	350^{0}C No reduction after 30 min at 170^{0}C	Water soluble so boiling and discarding the cooking water (e.g.in pasta) will reduce contamination

Sources: Kabak (2009), Stein and Bulboaca (2017), Tannous *et al.* 2016, Sobrova *et al.* 2010; Ryu *et al.* 2003

patulin by 90% through thermal processing are 105°C for 29 hours (Doyle *et al.* 1982). After such a treatment the patulin might have been denatured, but the apple juice is not likely to be very palatable. Normal HTST pasteurisation (90°C for 10 seconds) only reduced the patulin contamination by 18% (Wheeler *et al.* 1987) which is insufficient for a critical control point. Fermentation is reported to successfully reduce patulin in apple juice. Adding *Saccharomyces cerevisiae* (used in cider making) reduced patulin levels by 90% in three days (Doyle *et al.* 1982), although presumably there was a correlated increase in alcohol content, making it an unsuitable control method for small children and teetotallers. Roasting of nuts and coffee is often carried out for organoleptic reasons, and it has been shown to reduce aflatoxin levels in peanuts. Adding salt appears to enhance this degradation, but the reduction was only approximately 60% (Lee *et al.* 1969). Nixtamalisation is an alkaline cooking process used in tortilla production which is reported to reduce aflatoxin levels in the maize meal (Kabak 2008). In conclusion, thermal processes slightly reduce the mycotoxin levels, rather than eliminating the contamination, so they cannot be relied upon as single steps to ensure safety.

Excluding oxygen by vacuum packaging a food will inhibit aflatoxin production (Northolt and Bullerman 1982) but will not affect any toxin already produced.

Stein and Bubloaca (2017), Stoev (2013), Udomkun *et al.* (2017) and Patriarca and Pinto (2017) summarise various research papers which report on novel post-harvest processes and strategies to reduce or eliminate different mycotoxins in foods, including irradiation and chemical and biological agents to detoxify, extract, transform or inactivate the mycotoxins. However, all authors conclude that at present these methods are not sufficiently effective or practical for commercial application.

In summary, as most mycotoxins are heat stable and cannot be eliminated by currently available processing methods, the main control measure is to prevent or limit development in the food. This requires good agricultural practice, such as the protection of the crop from insect pests during growth and ripening, and rigorous post-harvest handling, including storage which is controlled for temperature and humidity and which protects from damage by pests. These post-harvest controls need to continue throughout the food chain.

Legislation and inspection

Many countries set legal standards for mycotoxins in food and feed. However, there is not universal agreement on accepted maximum levels. As an example, a Codex discussion paper (2017) on mycotoxins in spices included a summary of the different levels set by participating countries. For total aflatoxins in spices this ranges from 1 µ/kg in Honduras to 30 µ/kg in India, Pakistan and Sri Lanka. The EU sets 10 µ/kg and the US 20 µ/kg. There are a number of reasons why the maximum accepted levels may vary between countries, but if a food is being imported it must obviously comply with the legislation of the country receiving it, not the one sending it. Some of the foods which are known to be high risk for mycotoxins such as nuts, spices and dried fruit are imported into the EU from third countries where there may be lower standards. RASFF (2016) states that in the EU there were 418 border rejections and 82 alerts issued for mycotoxins in 2016. According to the same report, out of the top ten notifications, seven were for aflatoxins. Five of those were in nuts, nut products or seeds. One was in the category of herbs and spices and the other in fruit and vegetables. The significance of this contaminant is reflected in the additional controls that apply to the import of high risk products from particular countries under Commission Regulation (EU) No 884/2014. One of the requirements is that the products must be accompanied by certificates of analysis and a heath certificate signed by the competent authority in the exporting country. It should be noted that this certificate is only valid for four months from issue, since the toxins can develop during shipment and storage. Another requirement is that the products must enter through a Designated Point of Import (DPI). Noncompliance at import results in a border rejection. Noncompliance identified inland can result in seizure of the food and prosecution according to Commission Regulation (EC) 178/2002, article 14, placing food on the market which is unsafe.

Sampling

The determination of whether food stuff complies with the legal standards for mycotoxins set out in Commission Regulation (EC) No 1881/2006 requires a sample of the food stuff to be taken and analysed. Mycotoxins will *not* be homogeneously distributed through a foodstuff because of the way they are produced. A fungal spore is deposited on the food or plant, the fungus develops and mycotoxin may be produced by part of the fungal hyphae. This uneven distribution makes it a challenge to take a representative food sample. Taking one sample from a batch or lot may miss the contamination completely, or, if it was taken from a heavily contaminated section, may overestimate the mean level. To limit the impact of this problem, samples of food which are to be tested for mycotoxins must be aggregate samples. An aggregate sample is made up of a number of incremental samples, taken from various places in the food and mixed together. Commission Regulation (EC) No 401/2006 details the methods for sampling food for mycotoxins and defines both terms.

As a general rule, the larger the particle size of the food, the less evenly distributed the mycotoxin will be. Therefore as the particle size of the food increases, the sampling officer needs to take bigger (heavier) samples to ensure it is representative. This is to minimise the chance of missing a contaminated area or only sampling from a contaminated area. Either would be unrepresentative. Also, the number of incremental samples will need to increase as the overall amount of food gets larger. Happily the decisions about how much and how many incremental samples to take has been determined and published in Commission Regulation (EC) No 401/2006. The Regulation provides tables detailing the weight of the aggregate sample and the number of incremental samples required according to the foodstuff and the lot size (lot size being the overall quantity of food). One of the criteria for a DPI is that there are trained staff available to sample the products correctly, as it must be done according to Commission Regulation (EC) No 401/2006 to be meaningful.

The Food Standards Agency (2016) has produced guidance on the process of sampling for mycotoxins, giving additional advice on sampling at retail, and how to deal with pre-packed, scarce or lightweight products. In England, the Food Safety (Sampling and Qualifications) (England) Regulations 2013, Regulation 7 explains the procedure for taking any formal sample for analysis. This requires division of the sample into three parts, one of which should be presented to the owner of the food with notification that the sample is to be analysed. However, the Food Standards Agency (2016) guidance on sampling for mycotoxins (point 38) advises that, contrary to normal procedure (Anonymous 2017), when sampling for mycotoxins the officer should not divide into three parts at the point of sampling but take the entire aggregate sample to the analyst and allow the division into three parts to take place in the laboratory.

Future concerns

As more information becomes available on health impacts of various mycotoxins, organisations such as the WHO, EFSA and the FSA continue to evaluate the advice and controls. Two specific areas of focus are:

- The possibility of synergistic effects where more than one mycotoxin might be present in a food, at low levels.
- The possible impact of 'masked mycotoxins' where the toxins have been complexed to the food matrix. These may not be identified during sampling and analysis but could have a health impact when the food is digested.

Recent sampling indicated that cereal products on sale in the EU and in the US may be contaminated with more than one mycotoxin (Martins *et al.* 2018, Lee and Ryu 2015). Determining the potential health risk of low level ingestion of multiple mycotoxins is likely to be a complicated evaluation given the many options and diverse health effects that must be taken into account. EFSA is currently supporting projects which are developing models to help assess the impact of mixed mycotoxins. Hopefully these models will assist in re-evaluating the maximum accepted levels of contamination in food.

The effect of masked mycotoxins has also been the subject of recent research. Crews *et al.* (2016) report on in vitro studies which suggest that microbial activity in the human gut could enhance the release of free mycotoxins from masked mycotoxins in the food. The EFSA Panel on Contaminants in Food (CONTAM) has delivered a scientific opinion on the risks posed by masked mycotoxins, specifically the Fusarium toxins (zearalenone, nivalenol, T-2 and HT-2 toxins) (EFSA 2014). They expressed some concerns regarding zearalenone intake and, for toddlers and children, intake of fumonisins and modified fumonisins. However, in both studies the recommendations were to further investigate the subject, including the structure and analysis of these substances, the toxicology, animal health effects and any impact from processing in order to provide additional data for evaluation.

References

Abbas, H., W. Shier, J. Plasencia, M. Weaver, N. Bellaloui, J. Kotowiz, A. Butler, C. Accienelli, M. Eugenia de la Torre-Hernandez, R. Zablotowicz (2016); Mycotoxin contamination in corn smut (*Ustilago maydis*) galls in the field and in the commercial food products; *Food Control* 71:57–63

Abouzied M.M., A.D. Horvath, P.M. Podlesny, N.P. Regina, V.D. Metodiev, R.M. Kamenova-Tozeva, N.D. Niagolova, A.D. Stein, E.A. Petropoulos and V.S. Ganev (2002); Ochratoxin A concentrations in food and feed from a region with Balkan Endemic Nephropathy; *Food Additives & Contaminants* 19(8):755–64.

Alberts, J., W. van Zyl and W. Gelderblom (2016); Biologically based methods for control of Fumosin-producing Fusarium species and reductions of the Fumonisins; *Frontiers in Microbiology* 7; article 548:1–33

Anonymous (2017); Food Law Code of Practice (England); The Food Standards Agency https://www.food.gov.uk/sites/default/files/food_law_code_of_practice_2017.pdf accessed Nov 6 2017

Azziz-Baumgartner, E., K. Lindblade, K. Gieseker, H. Schurz Rogers, S. Kieszak, H. Njapau, R. Schleicher, L. McCoy, A. Misore, K. DeCock, C. Rubin and L. Slutsker (2005); Case control study of an acute aflatoxicosis outbreak, Kenya, 2004; *Environmental Health Perspectives* 113(12):1179–1783

Bennet, J.W. and M. Klich (2003); Mycotoxins; *Clinical Microbiology Reviews* 16(3):497–516

Codex Alimentarius (2017); Discussion paper on the establishment maximum levels for mycotoxins in spices; JOINT FAO/WHO FOOD STANDARDS PROGRAMME http://www.fao.org/fao-who-codexalimentarius/sh-proxy/es/?lnk=1andurl=https%253A%252F%252Fworkspace.fao.org%252Fsites%252Fcodex%252FMeetings%252FCX-735-11%252FWD%252Fcfl11_11e.pdf accessed Nov 8 2017

Crews, C., S. MacDonald, S. Gratz, S. Jones and A. Butler (2016); Masked mycotoxins in food and their release and uptake in the gut; FSA Final report available at https://www.food.gov.uk/sites/default/files/masked-mycotoxins-fs102101.pdf accessed October 25, 2017

Desjardins, A.E., T.M. Hohn and S.P. McCormick (1992); Effect of gene disruption of trichodiene synthase on the virulence of *Gibberella pulicaris*; *Molecular Plant-Microbe Interactions* 5(3):214–222

Dowd, P.F. (2001); Biotic and abiotic factors limiting efficacy of Bt Corn in indirectly reducing mycotoxin levels in commercial fields; *Journal of Economic Entomology* 94(5):1067–1074

Doyle, M.P., R.S. Applebaum; R.E. Brackett and E.H. Marth (1982); Physical, chemical and biological degradation of mycotoxins in foods and agricultural commodities; *Journal of Food Protection* 45(10):964–971

di Giuseppe, R., T. Bertuzzi, F. Rossi; S. Rastelli, A. Mulazzi; J. Capraro, A. de Curtis, L. Iacoviello, A. Pietri (2012); Plasma ochratoxin A levels, food consumption, and risk biomarkers of a representative sample of men and women from the Molise region in Italy; *European Journal of Nutrition* 51:851–860

Doster, M.A. and T.J. Michailides (1994); Development of *Aspergillus* molds in litter from pistachio trees; *Plant Disease* 78:393–397

Elling, F. and T. Moller (1973); Mycotoxic Nephropathy in Pigs; *Bulletin WHO* 79:411–418

EFSA (2014); Scientific opinion on the risks for human and animal health related to the presence of modified forms of certain mycotoxins in food and feed; *EFSA Journal* 12(12):3916 http://onlinelibrary.wiley.com/doi/10.2903/j.efsa.2014.3916/epdf

Food Standards Agency (2016); Mycotoxin Sampling Guidance https://www.food.gov.uk/sites/default/files/mycotoxins-sampling-guidance.pdf

FDA (2000); Guidance for Industry; https://www.fda.gov/Food/GuidanceRegulation/ucm077969.htm#afla

Geisen, R., N. Touhami and M. Schmidt-Heydt (2017); Mycotoxins as adaptation factors to food related environments; *Current Opinion in Food Science* 17:1–8

Georgiadou, M.A. Dimou and S. Yanniotis (2012); Aflatoxin contamination in pistachio nuts; *Food Control* 26:580–586

Kabak, B. (2008); The fate of mycotoxins during thermal food processing; *J Sci Food Agric* 89(4):549–554

Kabak, B. (2009); The fate of mycotoxins during thermal processing; *Journal of the Science of Food Agriculture* 89: 549–554

Kolliputi, V., R. Narasaiah, B. Sashidhar and C. Subramanyam (2006); Biochemical analysis of oxidative stress in the production of alflatoxin and its precursor intermediates; *Mycopathologia* 162:179–189

Kowalska, K., D. Habrowska-Górczy´ and A. Piastowska-Ciesielska (2016); Zearalenone as an endocrine disruptor in humans; *Environmental Toxicology and Pharmacology* 48:141–149

Krogh, P., B. Hald, R. Plestina and S. Ceovic (1977); Balkan (endemic) nephropathy and foodborne Ochratoxin A: Preliminary results of a survey of foodstuffs; *Acta Path et Microbiol Scand* Section B 85:238–240

International Agency for Research on Cancer (IARC) (2017); Agents classified by IARC Monographs volumes 1–119 http://monographs.iarc.fr/ENG/Classification/ accessed October 24, 2017

Lee, L.S., A.F. Cucullu, A.O. Franz and W.A. Pons (1969); Destruction of aflatoxins in peanuts during dry and oil roasting; *Journal of Agricultural and Food Chemistry* 17(3):451–453

Lee, H.J. and D. Ryu (2015); Advances in Mycotoxin Research: Public Health Perspectives; *Journal of Food Science* 80(12):T2970–T2983

Lewis, L., M. Onsongo, H. Njapau, H. Schurz Rogers. G. Luber, S. Kieszak, J. Nyamongo, L. Backer, A. Dahiye, A. Misore, K. DeCock and C. Rubin, (2005); Aflatoxin contamination of commercial maize products during an outbreak of acute aflatoxicosis in Eastern and Central Kenya; *Environmental Health Perspectives* 113(1):1763–1767

Malir, F., V. Ostry, A. Pfohl-Leszkowicz and E. Novotna (2013); Ochratoxin A: Developmental and reproductive toxicity—an overview; *Birth Defects Research (Part B)* 98:493–502

Martins, C., R. Assuncao, S. Cunha, J. Fernandes, A. Jager, T. Petta, C. Oliveira and P. Alvito (2018); Assessment of multiple mycotoxins in breakfast cereals available in the Portuguese market; *Food Chemistry* 239:132–140

Medina, A., A. Akbar, A. Baazeem, A. Rodriguez, and N. Magan (2017); Climate change, food security and mycotoxins: Do we know enough?; *Fungal Biology Reviews* 31:143–154

Misihairabgwi J.M., C.N. Ezekiel, M. Sulyok, G.S. Shephard and R. Krska (2017); Mycotoxin contamination of foods in Southern Africa: A 10-year review (2007–2016); *Critical Reviews in Food Science and Nutrition*, DOI: 10.1080/10408398.2017.1357003

Northolt, M. and L. Bullerman (1982); Prevention of mold growth and toxin production through control of environmental conditions; *Journal of Food Protection* 45(6):519–52

Ontario Ministry of Agriculture Food and Rural Affairs (OMAFRA) (2016); Patulin – a chemical concern for apple producers and processors; http://www.omafra.gov.on.ca/english/crops/facts/04-043.htm accessed November 6 2017

Patriarca, A. and Virginia Fernandez Pinto (2017); Prevalence of mycotoxins in foods and decontamination; *Current Opinion in Food Science* 14:50–60

Pitt, J.I. and J.D. Miller (2017); A concise history of mycotoxin research; *Journal of Agriculture and Food Chemistry* 65:7021–7033

RASFF (2016); Preliminary Report; European Commission Directorate-General For Health And Food Safety https://ec.europa.eu/food/sites/food/files/safety/docs/rasff_annual_report_2016.pdf

Rosner,H.; B. Rohrmann and G. Peiker (2000); Ochratoxin A in human serum; *Archiv für Lebensmittelhygiene* 51(4/5):104–107

Ross, R., J. Yuan, M. Yu, G. Wogan, G. Qian, J. Tu, J. Groopman, Y. Gao and B. Henderson (1992) Urinary aflatoxin biomarkers and risk of hepatocellular carcinoma; *Lancet* 339(8799):943–46

Ryu, D., M. Hanna, K. Eskridge and L. Bullerman (2003); Heat stability of zearalenone in an aqueous buffered model system; *Journal of Agriculture and Food Chemistry* 51(6):1746–1748

Sanzani, S.M., M. Reverberi, M. Punelli, A. Ippolito and C. Fanelli (2012); Study on the role of patulin on pathogenicity and virulence of *Penicillium expansum*; *International Journal of Food Microbiology* 153:323–331

Sobrova, P., V. Adam, A. Vasatkova, M. Beklova, L. Zeman and R. Kizek (2010); Deoxynivalenol and its toxicity; *Interdisciplinary Toxicology* 3(3):94–99.

Sommer, N.F., J.R. Buchanan and R.J. Fortlage (1986); Relation of early splitting and tattering of pistachio nuts to aflatoxin in the orchard; *Phytopathology* 76:692–694

Stein, R.A. and A.E. Bulboaca (2017); Chapter 21: Mycotoxins; In: *Foodborne Diseases*, 3rd edition, pp. 407–446; eds. Dodd C, T. Aldsworth and R. Stein; Academic Press

Stoev, S., D Goundasheva, T. Mirtcheva, and P.G. Mantle (2000); Susceptibility to secondary bacterial infections in growing pigs as an early response in Ochratoxicosis; *Experimental and Toxicologic Pathol*ogy 52(4):287–296.

Stoev, S. (2013); Food Safety and increasing hazard if mycotoxin occurrence in foods and feeds; *Critical reviews in Food Science and Nutrition* 53(9) 887–901

Swamy, H., T. Smith, N. Karrow and H.J. Boermans (2004); Effects of feeding blends of grains naturally contaminated with fusarium mycotoxins on growth and immunological parameters of broiler chickens; *Poultry Science* 83:533–543

Tannous, J., A. Atoui, A. El Khoury, Z. Francis, I. Oswald, O. Puel and R. Lteif (2016); A study on the physicochemical parameters for *Penicillium expansum* growth and patulin production: Effect of temperature, pH, and water activity; *Food Science and Nutrition* 4(4):611–622

Udomkun, P.; A.N. Wiredu, M. Nagle, J. Müller, B. Vanlauwe and R. Bandyopadhyay (2017); Innovative technologies to manage aflatoxins in foods and feeds and the profitability of application; *Food Control* 76:127–138

Wheeler, J.L., M.A. Harrison and P.E. Koehler (1987); Presence and stability of patulin in pasteurized apple cider; *Journal of Food Science* 52(2):479–480

WHO (1990); IPCS: Selected Mycotoxins; *Environmental Health Criteria* 105

Useful Websites

Triwood1973 (2009); How Pistachio Nuts Are Harvested and Processed; https://www.youtube.com/watch?v=qeJVTolV_KY accessed Sept 22 2017

TheFoodForest (2011); Pistachio Harvesting & Processing - Small Is Beautiful; https://www.youtube.com/watch?v=ABjHFy7u1Ek accessed Sept 22 2017

Ontario Ministry of Agriculture, Food and Rural Affairs (2016); Patulin - A Chemical Concern For Apple Producers & Processors; http://www.omafra.gov.on.ca/english/crops/facts/04-043.htm accessed March 12 2018

6   Parasites associated with meat

As with fish (discussed in Chapter 1), the significant parasites associated with meat belong to the Platyhelminthes and Nematoda. Meat undergoes a formal and rigorous process of inspection which helps control the public health impact of these parasites in the EU and other countries using these systems.

Platyhelminthes (flatworms)

The general comments contained in Chapter 1 about the Platyhelminthes also apply to those affecting meat. There are meat-associated examples from the same two parasitic classes, liver flukes (Trematoda) and tapeworms (Cestoda).

Trematoda (liver flukes)

One of the best known liver flukes associated with meat is *Fasciola hepatica*. Commonly called the sheep liver fluke, it is not species specific and can also inhabit cattle, humans and other mammals if the opportunity presents itself.

The intermediate host is a snail (normally *Lymnaea* [*Galba*] *truncatula* in the UK) which lives in damp boggy areas. Unusually for a trematode parasite from this subclass (Digenea), it has only one intermediate host. The metacercaria larvae, which must be ingested by the primary host for infestation, encysts externally on vegetation. Wet and flooded areas by rivers and streams are ideal. If a mammal eats the contaminated vegetation, the metacercaria will excyst in the intestines, migrate into the liver and develop into an adult liver fluke. A diagram of the lifecycle is shown in Figure 6.1. Sheep close crop grass, making them at serious risk of infestation which can impact significantly on their health. Infested animals suffer a range of symptoms as the parasites migrate through the gut wall to reach the liver. Once there, they burrow through the liver to reach the bile ducts. Symptoms include poor condition and failure to thrive, emaciation, liver damage and abscesses. An acute infestation can be fatal. The parasite has significant economic impact for sheep farmers (Kenyon *et al.* 2009). Farmers can treat infected animals with vermifuges, but there is increasing evidence that *Fasciola hepatica* is developing resistance to the drug of choice, triclabendazole. This drug affects the immature flukes rather than the adults. Treating the flukes before they reach

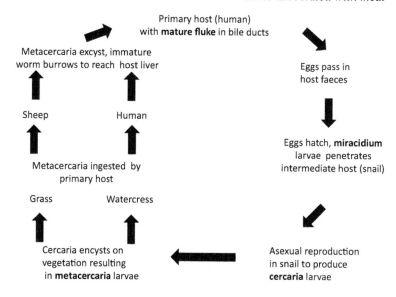

Figure 6.1 Life cycle of *Fasciola hepatica*

maturity minimises the damage to the sheep liver (Kelley *et al.* 2016). Cattle can also be infected, but the damage does not seem to be as extreme as in sheep (Mazeri *et al.* 2017).

Regulation EC 854/2004 specifies that sheep livers destined for human consumption must be palpated and incised to examine the bile ducts. Livers which show signs of infestation with *Fasciola hepatica* are discarded. The livers are often in poor condition from the damage caused by the liver flukes. Infested animals are not a risk for the food chain because eating the adult liver fluke would not cause infection in a human. Humans can be infected in a similar way to sheep, by directly chewing on contaminated vegetation. Once inside a human host, the flukes will take 3–4 months to reach maturity and can then live in the bile ducts for many years (Carnevale *et al.* 2016). A well-documented high risk food is water cress (Rondelaud *et al.* 2000). The cercaria larvae will attach to damp vegetation (to develop into the metacercaria), making water cress an ideal option. River banks and other wet areas adjacent to pasture where sheep graze will have a high risk for contamination. There is also evidence that rabbits and hares can act as the primary host (Rondelaud *et al.* 2001), continuing the infection of water cress beds even when the sheep are excluded. Cooking the water cress will destroy the larvae.

Changes in climate appear to be having an effect on the distribution of this parasite. The larval stages require a minimum temperature of 10°C, and both the intermediate host and free-living stages (miracidium and cercaria) need a moist environment. Increased rainfall and higher temperatures will enhance the transmission of *Fasciola hepatica,* and its appearance in areas such as south eastern

Scotland where it was previously unknown is being related to these changed weather patterns (Kenyon *et al.* 2009).

Cestoda (tapeworms)

This group has a number of meat associated parasites that can affect humans. The tapeworm is the adult form of the organism and inhabits the intestines of the primary host. The adult worm will have suckers and hooks on its head which are used to attach to the host intestine. The number and pattern on the hooks and suckers varies according to species but all have the same function – to anchor the head of the worm firmly while the body grows.

Like the liver flukes, these worms are dorsoventrally flattened but, unlike the trematodes, they can grow to considerable lengths. As the average human has approximately 23 feet of intestine, the worm has quite a lot of space in which to develop. Tapeworms absorb nutrients from the host gut contents. Nutrients are absorbed across the body wall or tegument, as tapeworms do not have a digestive system. Cestodes develop segmentally. The segments or proglottids develop from behind the miniscule head (the scolex) and enlarge as they mature. Mature segments containing fertilised eggs drop off the end of the worm and are excreted by the host in the faeces.

Cestodes associated with meat typically have two stages in the life cycle, the cystic stage, or bladder worm, and the adult tapeworm. The cystic stage (bladder worm) is usually found embedded in muscle or organs of a secondary host. The muscle (meat) of the secondary host must be eaten raw or undercooked by the primary host to cause infestation. Cooking destroys the bladder worm and is the most effective means of interrupting transmission.

When the primary host eats the undercooked infected muscle the bladder worm will be exposed to bile which is naturally excreted by the host into his/her small intestine. The bile causes the bladder worm to evaginate and mature, attaching its scolex into the intestinal wall. The bladder worm stage is typically given its own name by meat inspectors and veterinarians, which may cause confusion in the nomenclature. For example, 'Cysticercus bovis' is not a separate species but refers to the bladder worm stage of *Taenia saginata*.

Taenia saginata

The primary host for this parasite is humans. The intermediate host is the bovine, hence the name 'Cysticercus bovis' for the bladder worm stage. Infestation occurs when cattle eat *Taenia saginata* eggs which have contaminated their grazing or water supply. Once ingested, the larvae hatch and penetrate bovine gut. They use the bovine blood supply to reach the muscles where they encyst, forming a bladder worm or cysticercus. The cysts remain infective in the bovine for about ten weeks, after which they degenerate and calcify. If a human eats the meat raw or undercooked while the cysticeri are still viable, the cyst evaginates in the human gut, attaches and begins to develop and grow. Figure 6.2 shows a simplified life cycle of *Taenia saginata.*

In the EU, all beef must be inspected for Cysticercus bovis. The traditional way to do this is to focus the inspection on preferred places for the larvae to encyst such as the masseter muscles, heart and diaphragm. Regulation EC 854/2004 Annex I, section IV, chapter IX B defines meat infected with Cysticercus as unfit for human consumption but allows any uninfected parts of a carcass to be placed on the market after a suitable cold treatment to destroy the bladder worms. These uninfected parts must be frozen for three weeks at -7°C or two weeks at -10°C (Wilson 1998, Regulation EC 854/2004). The beef is then considered safe to eat. There are limitations in the meat inspection process. Viable cysts are less conspicuous than calcified cysts and may not be identified. Lightly infected animals are more likely to be missed by inspectors as there will be fewer cysts and these might not be at the site of incision. Researchers have tried to evaluate the sensitivity of meat inspection for identifying Cysticercus bovis. Dorny *et al.* (2000) used serological tests (ELISA) to determine the prevalence of Cysticercus bovis in 1164 cattle from 20 abattoirs. The blood testing indicated that the inspectors were only identifying 10% of the contaminated carcasses. The others were passed as fit for human consumption.

The contamination rate in cows in the EU is considered to be low, even allowing for the low sensitivity of the meat inspection process. For example, in the period 2011–2013, Belgium reported 0.12–0.16% of slaughtered carcasses were contaminated (EFSA 2015), and in France in 2010 it was 0.14% (Dupuy *et al.* 2014). Rates in the UK are considered to be of the same order of magnitude

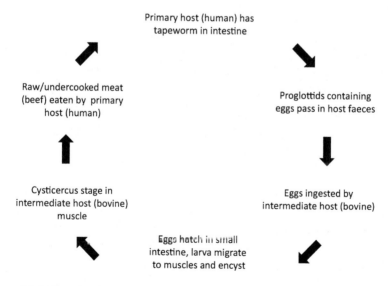

Figure 6.2 Life cycle of *Taenia saginata*

(Marshall *et al.* 2015). This low incidence is mainly due to the correct disposal of human sewage. Separating raw human waste from farm land interrupts the life cycle by preventing the cows from ingesting the fertilised eggs. Not all sewage treatment processes destroy *Taenia saginata* eggs, so if sewage sludge is to be spread on pastures, there should be at least a six month gap before cows are allowed onto the pasture to minimise the chance of infection. Effluent from sewage works can also contaminate the watercourses from which cows drink and Cabaret *et al.* (2002) suggest this is a more important mechanism of infection than sludge spreading, in part because sludge spreading is uncommon on pastures in the EU and because where it does happen it is highly regulated (Dupuy *et al.* 2014). However, the importance of the connection between human sewage and bovine infection should not be overlooked and is demonstrated by a slightly unusual incident reported in 2013. In a batch of cows presented for slaughter at a UK abattoir, a remarkable 70% were positive for Cysticercus bovis. On investigation it was found that cattle from other farms (five in total) were also infested. There were two possible sources of the infection. Both items had been fed to the affected cows. One possible source was oilseed rape straw that had been grown on land fertilised with human sewage. The other was potatoes which had been transported by road from continental Europe. The potatoes were originally intended for human consumption, but downgraded on arrival to animal feed when it was discovered that illegal immigrants had travelled with the potatoes and contaminated them with human faeces during the journey (Featherstone *et al.* n.d.; DEFRA 2015). Some non–EU countries report higher contamination rates than in Europe, for example 5.2% of cattle slaughtered between May and June 2014 in an abattoir in Northern Ethiopia (Belay and Mekelle 2014) and 6.09% of cattle slaughtered January–December 2015 in Menofia, Egypt (Elkhtam *et al.* 2016) were positive for Cysticercus bovis.

In the UK, DEFRA report a low level of human cases (Table 6.1). However, *Taenia saginata* is not a notifiable disease, so the incidence may be higher. The species of tapeworm in the DEFRA reports is not specified and the notifications could be fish related (Chapter 1) as well as meat associated (see DEFRA annual zoonoses reports available online) but Hill *et al.* (2013) state that 98% of the reports in 2011 were *Taenia saginata*. Some, at least, of the infections are considered to have been acquired abroad. Given that meat inspection reduces, rather than eliminates, the risk that Cysticercus bovis contaminated meat will reach the consumer, the most effective way to prevent human infection is to ensure all beef is thoroughly cooked. Raw beef such as carpaccio, rare beef (steaks, roasts) and fermented beef sausages can all act as sources of human infection and probably account for the cases identified in the UK annually (Table 6.1). Food business operators wishing to produce or serve raw or rare beef can freeze it for two weeks prior to use. This will eliminate any cysts without affecting the eating quality of the meat. Human infections are usually considered by the medical profession to be of low impact and are often asymptomatic. The patient may be unaware of the infestation unless the proglottids are observed in the faeces. In a heroic effort to push the boundaries of science, a volunteer self-infected with two Cysticercus

Table 6.1 Notifications of human parasite infections

Year	Taenia in UK	Echinococcosis in UK			Trichinellosis in EU
		No. cases	Associated with sheep	Indigenous	
2001	107				53
2002	75				48
2003	87				97
2004	92				270
2005	72	11	0	0	175
2006	87	14	0	0	706
2007	98	10	0	0	780
2008	99	18	0	0	670
2009	73	9	0	0	750
2010	112	7	2	2	223
2011	94	15	0	0	268
2012	70	6	0	0	301*
2013	79	14	0	0	217*
2014	70	16	0	0	320*
2015	85	16	0	0	–

(Alban *et al.* 2011; DEFRA 2007–2017; ECDC 2010–2015b)

*laboratory confirmed

bovis cysts, observed the results for six months and then published these observations (Tembo and Craig 2015). Apart from some sporadic diarrhoea, the main symptom appeared to be 'painless involuntary rectal sensations' 11–12 weeks after infection which coincided with the appearance of the proglottids in the faeces. The infection is common in sub-Saharan Africa and the Middle East, and there were an estimated 60 million cases worldwide in 1992 (Raether and Hanel 2003). The WHO (2017) claims that *Taenia saginata* does not impact on human health in any significant way. However most consumers would probably prefer not to host a parasitic tapeworm and in patients already suffering from poor nutrition or ill health, a long-term infection would seem unlikely to improve their situation.

Taenia solium

The primary host for *Taenia solium* is also a human being. As with *Taenia saginata*, the adult tapeworm forms in the human intestine. The intermediate host for *Taenia solium* is a pig. The bladder worm (cystic) stage for *Taenia solium* is known as Cysticercus cellulosae, and the typical life cycle is very similar to that of *Taenia saginata* in that the secondary host (pig) ingests eggs that have been excreted by the human host, the eggs cross the intestinal wall and use the blood supply to reach the muscles. A process of development or maturation results in bladder worms (cysticerci) forming in the pig muscle. The next primary host is infected by eating undercooked or raw pork. Figure 6.3 shows a simplified life cycle.

In the UK, pig carcasses with Cysticercus cellulosae are rejected by inspectors. There have been no reports of cysts in pigs in UK for some time (DEFRA 2008), making it now quite a rare parasite. The low incidence in the UK is mainly due to the way in which pigs are reared for human consumption. Most pigs are reared intensively, in controlled industrial settings. The animals are highly managed with customised housing, controlled access to outdoor spaces and commercially produced food. Even farms which produce outdoor reared pigs tend to be part of a quality assurance scheme (Hill *et al.* 2013) which ensures good hygiene and a controlled food supply. As a consequence, in the UK, the chance of pigs coming into contact with human faeces containing *Taenia solium* eggs is negligible. Consumers may have some concerns regarding animal welfare in an indoor, intensive pig rearing system (Thorslund *et al.* 2017), but there is no doubt that it serves to interrupt the life cycle of *Taenium solium* very satisfactorily.

This is fortunate because, in contrast to *Taenia saginata,* there is the potential for serious health impact from this parasite. Infestation with the adult tapeworm (i.e. becoming the primary host by eating raw or rare pork) is considered to be no more problematic than being infected with the bovine tapeworm, *Taenia saginata* (WHO 2017, Garcia *et al.* 2003) and infected people are usually asymptomatic (Laranjo-González *et al.* 2017). However, humans can act as either primary or secondary host to *Taenia solium*, and being the secondary host has more serious consequences. If a human ingests viable eggs from *Taenia solium,* the eggs will develop in the same way they do in the pig, that is to say the gastric fluids will initiate development of the eggs into larvae which encyst in the human host. If this

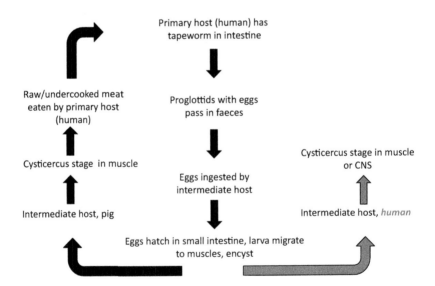

Figure 6.3 Life cycle of *Taenia solium*

happens in host striated muscle, small nodules develop which can become tender and inflamed but eventually degenerate. They may calcify but do not appear to cause major health impact. The real problem is if the bladder worms encyst on the central nervous system (CNS) causing neurocysticercosis (NCC) (WHO 2017). This can result in epileptic seizures (50–80% of cases), intracranial hypertension and/or hydrocephalus (both in 20–30% of cases) (Garcia *et al.* 2003). All of these can be fatal. There is also a possibility that the parasites can encyst in the patients' eyes causing ophthalmic cysticercosis. This is rare, occurring in 1–3% of cases (Garcia *et al.* 2003). The WHO (2017) estimates that 2.56–8.30 million people worldwide suffer from neurocysticercosis as a result of infection with eggs from *Taenia solium.*

Humans only become infested with the cystic form of *Taenia solium* (Cycsticercus cellulosae) by ingesting the fertilised eggs. One obvious way is to eat food contaminated by a food handler who hosts a tapeworm. The food does not have to be pork – it can be any ready-to-eat food contaminated directly or indirectly. Schantz *et al.* (1992) report on four unrelated people in New York who were diagnosed with NCC following seizures. Screening of family contacts identified two more people with cystic lesions and seven with antibodies for cycsticerci. All the patients and their families were Orthodox Jews who had no contact with pork. However, one of their domestic staff (from Latin America) was hosting *Taenia solium* and another was serologically positive. Hira *et al.* (2004) report a similar situation from Kuwait. There are no pigs or pork products in the country, but nine Kuwaitis developed NCC which was acquired in Kuwait. Screening identified a cook from an endemic country who had positive antibodies for *Taenia solium.* There are also reports of autochthonous infection from Qatar (Khan *et al.* 2011) and Saudi Arabia (Al Shahrani *et al.* 2003). The most plausible explanation in these cases is cross-contamination of ready-to-eat food by infected food handlers with poor hygiene.

Laranjo-González *et al.* (2017) carried out a systematic review of all published reports of human cyctercercosis in Western Europe between 1990 and 2015. They found case reports in 16 EU member states (including the UK) and Switzerland. Del Brutto (2012) carried out a similar review for the period 1970–2011 and found that the cases of human cycticercosis steadily increased in the EU over that period. It should be noted that these are absolute numbers, not corrected for population, so the incidence may not be increasing. However, he also found that the type of patient is changing. In the earlier decades, the disease was associated with older patients living in villages where pigs were reared in traditional ways for home consumption. These are well known risk factors, under good control in most parts of the EU. The later cases were younger people living in urban areas. Some were immigrants or EU citizens who had travelled to areas where *Taenia solium* is endemic, but there were also what appear to be autochthonous cases in EU citizens. As there is practically no porcine cycticercosis reported in most EU countries, and, where there is, it is often associated with small production for home/local use (Zammarchi *et al.* 2013), there is clearly some other reason for the change in disease profile and a possible change in prevalence. The number of cases in the EU does appear to be quite low. Del Brutto (2012) identified that Portugal and Spain had the highest number of reported cases over the study period 1970–2011 (384 and 228 respectively). The UK was fourth with 26, behind France with 80. Neither *Taenia solium* nor cysticercosis are notifiable in the EU and researchers have had to rely on publications which report incidents. As a consequence, it is likely that many cases are undiagnosed and/or unreported. The real numbers are likely to be higher. Cysticercosis is considered to be an increasing problem in the US as well as the EU. To evaluate the problem O'Keefe *et al.* (2015) looked at hospital notifications in the USA during 1998–2011. They report a hospitalisation rate of approximately 8 per one million people over that period and suggest the disease burden may be underestimated in the USA.

A human with cysticercosis represents a stop in the life cycle of the parasite. Although the impact of the disease can be significant, indeed fatal, for the patient, a person with cysticercosis cannot pass it on. Infection has to be acquired from a human with the tapeworm. The prevalence of home acquired *Taenia solium* in the EU is unclear as it is difficult to distinguish between *Taenia solium* and *Taenia saginata.* However, given the lack of porcine cysticercosis in the EU it is likely to be a very low number. Laranjo-González *et al.* (2017) were able to identify confirmed reports of only 22 cases of *Taenia solium* between 1990 and 2015 in the EU although the sales of anti-helminth drugs suggest the prevalence of Taeniosis is much higher. Researchers consider that the increase in human cysticercosis in the US and the EU, and its appearance in Muslim countries like Kuwait, reflects the movement of human carriers from endemic areas who are already infected with *Taenia solium.* These carriers excrete the ripe proglottids and the eggs are somehow ingested by other people in the vicinity. In the US and Spain, the main source of the carriers is considered to be Latin America (Del Brutto 2012, O'Keefe *et al.* 2015), in France and Portugal it is thought that people from sub-Saharan Africa may be contributing and in the UK the source appears mainly to be India (Del Brutto 2012).

The movement of people from endemic areas into controlled areas can increase the risk of human cysticercosis in the controlled areas, especially if they are employed as food handlers. The eggs of *Taenia solium* are infectious as soon as they are deposited, and each egg can develop into an adult tapeworm. After defecation the hosts can carry the eggs under their fingernails and on their skin and clothes. This makes it easy to contaminate ready-to-eat food. *Taenia solium* can be long lived in a human host (up to 25 years according to Hoberg 2002), producing 50,000 eggs per proglottid which can be shed at the rate of 6 per day (CDC 2013), so a single carrier can cause widespread infection for long periods. Given the difficulty in assessing the extent of the problem, most researchers suggest that cases of both *Taenia solium* and cysticercosis (human and porcine) should be notifiable. In some American states (Arizona, California, New Mexico, Oregon, Texas and Alaska), notification is already required (O'Keefe *et al.* 2015). Universal requirement for notification would assist in establishing the extent of the problem and whether it is increasing, decreasing or remaining stable. It would also raise awareness in the medical profession where underdiagnoses appear to be an issue (Zammarchi *et al.* 2013). Screening programmes have been suggested to identify carriers of *Taenia solium*. Microscopic examination of faecal samples is the classic method. Unfortunately, because the eggs are not uniformly shed in the faeces, this test is not very sensitive, risking false negatives, and it is not usually possible to distinguish between the eggs of *Taenia solium* and *Taenia saginata*. ELISA assay for tapeworm antigens in the faecal sample is a better option (Gilman *et al.* 2012). Recombinant enzyme-linked immunoelectrotransfer blot (EITB rES33) can identify *Taenia solium* in blood samples but does not distinguish between previous and current infection (O'Neal et al. 2014). According to Gabriël *et al.* (2013), Greece is the only EU country that currently screens immigrants for *Taenia solium* (method not stated). The CDC (2011) does not recommend screening food handlers, only household employees where there has been a confirmed diagnosis of NCC. Routine screening of food handlers for faecal pathogens has become unpopular in the UK. It is viewed as an intrusive and expensive process which provides limited information since it can only confirm the handler's health on the day of screening. This is correct for enteric bacteria like *Salmonella* where the handler can be infected at any time after screening. However, in the case of *Taenia solium*, a negative sample should remain negative unless the handler revisits the endemic area. It is very unlikely he or she could be infected here in the UK.

The Food Standards Agency (2009), in its Guidance on Fitness to Work, recommends that food handlers suffering with *Taenia solium* should be excluded from handling open and ready-to-eat foods pending two consecutive clear stool samples. The document also states that the organism is rare in the UK. In fact, its true prevalence is unknown. The food industry in the UK is extremely multicultural and it would probably be helpful if more detailed guidance was given on this particular parasite, especially for food business operators who have staff moving between endemic areas and the UK. People hosting *Taenia solium* are typically asymptomatic and so unlikely to demonstrate any of the health problems listed in annex 3 of the Guidance, which is recommended for use to establish fitness to work.

Thorough handwashing is the intervention used to prevent infection through the faecal oral route and this is recommended to control human cysticercosis (Meštrovic *et al.* 2012, CDC 2013). However, there do not appear to be any studies on the impact of hand washing on the transmission of this parasite. It seems to be assumed that it will be efficacious. Given the fact that eggs have been isolated from under the fingernails of hosts, handwashing will need to be very thorough to prevent an infected food handler causing significant cysticercosis if s/he is preparing ready-to-eat food. Several researchers have identified human cysticercosis as an emerging hazard in the EU due to increased tourism into, and migration out from, endemic areas (EFSA 2000, Del Brutto 2013, Devleesschauwer *et al.* 2017, Laranjo-González *et al.* 2017). However all the current monitoring seems focused on reporting incidents in animals (Dorny *et al.* 2010, EFSA 2016, Devleelsschauwer *et al.* 2017) rather than tracking the human carriers of the adult tapeworm. It is quite possible that this is an emerging pathogen and one which could have serious public health impact.

Echinococcus granulosus

Echinococcus granulosus causes hydatid disease or echinococcosis and differs from the other two tapeworms described here in that the adult is very small. The primary host for *Echinococcus granulosus* is a dog. There can be several intermediate hosts – sheep is the most common, but also pigs, cattle and humans can also be infected.

The eggs of *Echinococcus granulosus* need to be ingested by an intermediate host (Figure 6.4). As with the cystic stage of *Taenia solium*, this usually means eating food contaminated directly or indirectly with faeces, but in this case it is dog faeces, rather than human. Cases are also reported of people failing to wash their hands between handling their dogs and eating some food and ingesting the eggs in that way. Once inside the sheep (or human) the embryos will penetrate the wall of the intestine and spread to the host's organs – typically the liver, but also the lungs, kidney, spleen and heart. Cysts then develop on the organs.

In humans, about 70% of infections involve cystic lesions on the liver (Wang *et al.* 2008) but other organs may be involved. Ahmadi and Hamidi (2008) report that the lungs are the second most common organ affected in human echinococcosis, although lung cysts are more commonly associated with a related organism, *Echinococcus multilocularis*. *Echinococcus multilocularis* has a similar lifecycle and is apparently much more serious if transmitted to humans. In a two-year period of surveillance in Europe (1998–2000), Kern *et al.* (2003) report the death of over 20% of the patients presenting with symptoms. They consider that the alveolar echinoccocus was definitely responsible for death in 10.9% of the patients and probably responsible in another 12.6%. However, *Echinococcus multilocularis* is associated with foxes and other small mammals rather than food animals and therefore not considered food related (DEFRA 2008). Treatment of echinococcosis is usually by surgery.

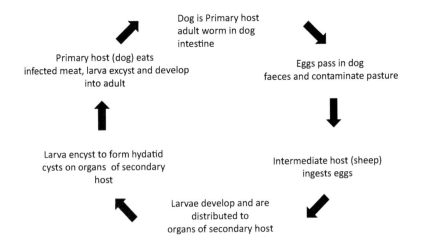

Figure 6.4 Life cycle of *Echinococcus granulosus*

Human victims do not generally acquire either species of the echinococcus parasite from eating raw infected meat but by ingesting the eggs which have been excreted by the primary host (i.e. ingesting dog faeces, presumably indirectly). However, meat species such as sheep, pigs and cattle may be infected as intermediate hosts, and the affected organs should not be used for human consumption.

The prevalence of the disease in humans varies. In some countries it is endemic and a high proportion of the population are affected. The WHO (2008) estimates, for example, that 6.6% of the population in the Tibetan Plateau are infected. Proximity to dogs and a rural lifestyle are risk factors (Ahmadi and Hamidi 2008, WHO 2008, Wang *et al.* 2008). In urbanised areas such as the majority of the EU this risk is reduced. Notifications in the EU range from 486 in 1995 to 374 in 2003 with a high of 592 in 1996.This may well include cases of *Echinococcus multilocularis* as the species is not always determined. As with other parasites, the accession of new member states has increased the notifications of *Echinococcus*. In 2008 there were 911 cases reported in the EU. These were not evenly spread. Many countries report none or very few cases, while Bulgaria had the highest notification rate, accounting for 386 notifications or 5 per 100,000 of population (ECDC 2010).

In the UK in 1999 there were two cases associated with sheep farming. From 2000 onwards DEFRA (2006, 2007, 2008) report no cases had an association with sheep farming until 2010. There are none reported since then (Table 6.1). Foxes can also act as primary host but their contribution to the human disease statistics is unknown.

Nematoa (round worms)

Round worms are small worms with very little differentiation that is immediately obvious to the naked eye. They are slim and elongate with pointed ends and a complex cuticle which provides good protection from the environment. They require water in which to move and do not appear to have the armoury of unpleasant hooks and suckers exhibited by the flatworms. The general comments made in Chapter 1 about nematodes also apply here.

Trichinella spiralis

The main nematode parasite associated with meat is *Trichinella spiralis*. Both the primary and secondary host are mammals, and the organism is not species specific. In the primary host (which can include pig, rat, dog, horse, human) the adult worm inhabits the intestines. In the intermediate host (which include the same species as the primary host) the larvae encyst in the muscles (Figure 6.5). The infestation happens in the following manner:

- a mammal eats infected meat raw
- the host gastric juices trigger excysting of the larvae

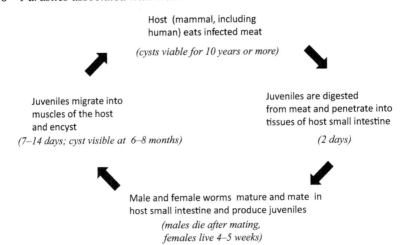

Host (mammal, including
human) eats infected meat

(cysts viable for 10 years or more)

Juveniles migrate into
muscles of the host
and encyst
(7–14 days; cyst visible at 6–8 months)

Juveniles are digested
from meat and penetrate into
tissues of host small intestine
(2 days)

Male and female worms mature and mate in
host small intestine and produce juveniles
(males die after mating,
females live 4–5 weeks)

Figure 6.5 Life cycle of *Trichinella*

- adult worms mature and live in the small intestine often causing diarrhoea and abdominal pain (1–2 weeks)
- eggs are deposited in lymph spaces
- the larvae develop and migrate into blood, possibly accompanied by flu- like symptoms and /or fever
- the larvae spread to muscles, usually causing myalgia /rheumatism like pains
- larvae remain encysted until eaten.

The best control mechanism for this parasite is to ensure thorough cooking of all raw meat. However, some meat products such as fermented sausages and traditional hams will contain uncooked meat and will be eaten in that state. These products can cause infection if made from infected meat. Heavily salted, smoked and dried hams can be made safe using a hurdle technique by curing for 40 days, followed by smoking at 45°C for ten days (Gracey 1981).

Under Regulation EC 854/2004, Annex I, Section IV, Chapter IX C, meat from animals infected with *Trichinella spiralis* is considered unfit for human consumption. Visual inspection, palpation and incision do not identify *Trichinella spiralis*. It is possible to inspect carcasses for the cysts using microscopy (a trichinoscope). However, this is not very fast (3–6 min per sample) or efficient. An alternate is the digestion test where the muscle to be tested is dissolved using pepsin and hydrochloric acid (HCl), and any cysts then examined under microscope.

Trichinella spiralis is mainly associated with temperate regions of the world. There have been no human cases associated with UK-produced meat since 1975 (DEFRA 2007). However, in the period 1975–2006 there have been 39 laboratory confirmed cases in humans in the UK, but all are believed to have been acquired abroad or from imported meat (DEFRA 2007). There have been no cases reported in the UK in 2006–2009, but in 2010 a case associated with French-produced meat was reported (DEFRA 2008, 2009, 2010). There were no cases reported in 2011, 2012 or 2013. Since 1999 the UK had monitored wildlife (foxes, badgers and various birds) for *Trichinella* infestation. However, this programme ended in March 2015 as the samples were consistently negative (DEFRA 2017). There has been only one recent outbreak reported in the UK (eight cases in 2000). This was associated with imported food.

There are reports of human cases in other EU member states. These are mainly sporadic cases, but outbreaks have been recorded in Spain (Gomez-Garcia *et al.* 2003), Bulgaria, Estonia, France, Germany, Greece, Hungary, Italy, Latvia, Lithuania, Poland, Romania and Slovakia (Alban *et al.* 2011). Infection in the EU is often associated with game such as wild boar meat, which will generally not have been inspected, or home killed uninspected pork (Anonymous 2003). A recent incident in Germany illustrates the risk. Some meat from wild boar was made into cured sausages (8 kg) and the remains (30–35 kg) were sold for roasting. Seventy-one people who ate the meat were subsequently confirmed as having trichinellosis. All those who ate sausages ate them raw. How the roast was cooked is not reported. Tests on some of the remaining sausages indicated a larval contamination rate of 0.3 to 0.7 larvae per gram (Faber *et al.* 2015). Making fermented sausages which are designed to be eaten raw, from meat which has been reared under controlled conditions and properly inspected, reduces the risk of parasitism. Doing the same thing with uninspected wild game is a very high risk process and likely to cause illness.

The increase in trichinellosis notifications indicated in Table 6.1 coincides with the two major expansions of the EU. In the first expansion (2004), the population from which notifications were received increased, and as these are absolute numbers, not corrected per head of population, it was unsurprising that total notifications increased as well. It should be noted that some of the acceding states such as Cyprus were free of *Trichinella*. The second expansion again increased the population but included states such as Romania and Bulgaria which have high notifications of the disease by comparison with the UK. More recent data appears to show a drop in notifications. According to the European Centre for Disease Prevention and Control (ECDC), the rate of infection 2010–2014 varies between 0.05 and 0.07 per 100,000 population, but Romania and Bulgaria still make significant contribution to the incidence (ECDC 2015a and 2015b). It is probably unwise to source pork from these areas if it is to be used in fermented sausage or other products which will not undergo heat treatment.

Meat inspection

Meat inspection is carried out in slaughter houses by veterinarians and meat Inspectors. The *post mortem* meat inspection processes are detailed in Regulation EC 854/2004 and involve visual inspection, palpation and incision of specified parts of the carcass and organs. The main objective is to protect public health by identifying animals with signs of zoonoses. Every carcass and organ is individually inspected. These procedures are historic and were developed to prevent diseases that are now rare. The main reason for their rarity is that animals for slaughter in the UK and most of the EU now tend to be reared in controlled conditions with veterinary interventions and extensive use of quality assurance systems. This results in herds which are very consistent and protected from exposure. The main hazards now associated with meat are those which cannot be identified by visual inspection, palpation or incision, such as contamination with *Salmonella* or pathogenic *E. coli*. There is some suggestion that the process of meat inspection itself may act to enhance these microbial hazards by cross contamination (EFSA 2011) but the evidence is not conclusive (Hill *et al.* 2013). As traditional *post mortem* meat inspection is labour intensive, expensive and not actually addressing the main hazards, the European Commission supports the development of more risk based inspection rather than spending scarce resources looking for something that is not there, such as *Cysticercus cellulosae* in indoor reared pigs. The first stage of this development is a move away from visual inspection, palpation and incision for all animals to visual inspection only for those which meet controlled conditions of rearing (EC 2000). This option has always been permitted under Regulation EC 854/2004 but infrequently used. The Food Standards Agency has funded research to evaluate what the impact of visual only inspection might have on public health. The conclusion from these risk assessments was that for pigs, sheep, goats and wild/farmed deer the increased risk to public health would be negligible. However, the researchers estimate there could be an increased risk of approximately 20% for contracting *Taenia saginata* from beef that has undergone visual only inspection (Hill *et al.* 2013, Hill *et al.* 2014). It should be emphasised that visual only inspection would apply when the animals meet predetermined criteria such as the supply of full food chain information and compliance with controlled rearing conditions. Animals would still undergo full inspection if the ante-mortem inspection, the food chain information or any other indicator suggested it might be necessary.

Wild meat that has not been properly inspected and is eaten rare carries a high risk of causing infection. In Ohio in 1998, eight people developed trichinosis. This was attributed to eating Canadian bear meat which had been made into burgers and barbequed but eaten rare (Nelson *et al.* 2003). Cases of trichinosis are also reported in China (Liu and Boireau 2002) where between 1980–1989 there were 15,599 cases and 141 deaths from the organism. These figures correlated with increased economic prosperity in 20 provinces, which resulted in increased meat consumption by the inhabitants. It was estimated that 94.3% of the cases were caused by eating raw or undercooked pork and the remainder by eating dog.

Good husbandry and meat inspection have reduced the incidence of trichinosis in many countries. This is an important intervention. An outbreak reported in Serbia in December 2001–January 2002 involved 309 people who had eaten smoked sausages made by a commercial meat processor. The investigation identified a number of failures including poor inspection processes. The investigators claim the political, economic and demographic changes which occurred as a result of the civil war contributed to the outbreak. Many of the experienced veterinarians had apparently moved away, so proper meat inspection processes did not take place. The large controlled abattoirs with in-house inspectors closed during the upheaval and were replaced with many small abattoirs unable to provide proper continuous inspection. A re-emergence of trichinosis resulted (Djordjevic *et al.* 2003).

References

Ahmadi N.A. and M. Hamidi (2008); A retrospective analysis of human cystic echinococcosis in Hamedan province, an endemic region of Iran; *Annals of Tropical Medicine and Parasitology* 102(7):603–609

Alban, L., E. Pozio, J. Boes, P. Boireau, F. Boué, M. Claes, A.J.C. Cook, P. Dorny, H.L. Enemark, J. van der Giesseng, K.R. Hunt, M. Howell, M. Kirjusina, K. Nöckler, P. Rossi, G.C. Smith, L. Snow, M.A. Taylor, G. Theodoropoulos, I. Vallée, M.M. Viera-Pinto, I.A. Zimmer (2011); Towards a standardised surveillance for *Trichinella* in the European Union; *Preventive Veterinary Medicine* 99(2011):148–160

Al Shahrani, D., H. Frayha, O. Dabbagh, E. Al Shail (2003); First case of Neurocysticercosis in Saudi Arabia, *Journal of Tropical Pediatrics* 49(1):58–60

Anonymous (2003); Report of trends and sources of zoonotic agents in the EU and Norway; SANCO/339/2005 Part 1 http://ec.europa.eu/food/food/biosafety/salmonella/09_echinococcus_2003.pdf

Belay, S. and A. Mekelle (2014); Prevalence of Cysticercus bovis in cattle at municipal abbatoir of Shire; *Journal of Veterinary Science and Technology* 5:4

Carnevale, S., J.B. Malandrini, M.L. Pantano, M. Sawicki, C.C. Soria, L.H. Kuo and J.N. Velásquez (2016); *Fasciola hepatica* infection in humans: Overcoming problems for the diagnosis; *Acta Parasitologica* 61(4):776–783

Cabaret, J., S. Geerts, M. Madeline, C. Ballandonne and D. Barbier (2002); The use of urban sewage sludge on pastures: The cysticercosis threat; *Vet Res* 33:575–597

CDC (2011); Taeniasis; Resources for health professionals; https://www.cdc.gov/parasites/cysticercosis/health_professionals/index.html accessed November 18 2017

CDC (2013); Taeniasis; https://www.cdc.gov/parasites/taeniasis/biology.html accessed November 18 2017

DEFRA (2007) Zoonoses UK Annual Report; http://webarchive.nationalarchives.gov.uk/20110318141136/http://www.defra.gov.uk/foodfarm/farmanimal/diseases/atoz/zoonoses/documents/reports/zoonoses2007.pdf accessed March 29, 2018

DEFRA (2008) Zoonoses UK Annual Report; http://webarchive.nationalarchives.gov.uk/20110318141134/http://www.defra.gov.uk/foodfarm/farmanimal/diseases/atoz/zoonoses/documents/report-2008.pdf accessed March 29, 2018

DEFRA (2009) Zoonoses UK Annual Report; https://www.gov.uk/government/uploads/system/uploads/attachment_data/file/69313/pb13571-zoonoses2009-110125.pdf accessed March 29, 2018

DEFRA (2010) Zoonoses UK Annual Report; https://www.gov.uk/government/uploads/system/uploads/attachment data/file/69315/pb13627-zoonoses-report2010.pdf accessed March 29, 2018

DEFRA (2011) Zoonoses UK Annual Report; https://www.gov.uk/government/uploads/system/uploads/attachment_data/file/69638/pb13851-zoonoses-2011.pdf accessed March 29, 2018

DEFRA (2012) Zoonoses UK Annual Report; https://www.gov.uk/government/uploads/system/uploads/attachment_data/file/236983/pb13987-zoonoses-report-2012.pdf accessed March 29, 2018

DEFRA (2013) Zoonoses UK Annual Report; https://www.gov.uk/government/uploads/system/uploads/attachment_data/file/447771/pb13987-zoonoses-report-2013.pdf accessed March 29, 2018

DEFRA (2014) Zoonoses UK Annual Report; https://www.gov.uk/government/uploads/system/uploads/attachment_data/file/621686/zoonoses-annual-report-2014.pdf accessed March 29, 2018

DEFRA (2015) Zoonoses UK Annual Report; https://www.gov.uk/government/uploads/system/uploads/attachment_data/file/621094/UK_Zoonoses_report_2015.pdf accessed March 29, 2018

DEFRA (2016) Zoonoses UK Annual Report; https://www.gov.uk/government/uploads/system/uploads/attachment_data/file/664448/UK_Zoonoses_report_2016.pdf accessed March 29, 2018

DEFRA (2017); Zoonoses Report UK 2015; DEFRA; https://www.gov.uk/government/uploads/system/uploads/attachment_data/file/621094/UK_Zoonoses_report_2015.pdf accessed March 15 2018

Del Brutto, O.H. (2012); Neurocysticercosis in Western Europe: A re-emerging disease?; *Acta Neurologica Belgica* 112:335–343

Del Brutto, O.H. (2013); Neurocysticercosis: New thoughts on controversial issues; *Current Opinion in Neurology 2013* 26:289–294

Devleesschauwer, B., A. Allepuz, V. Dermauw, M. Johansen, M. Laranjo-González, G. Smit, S. Sotiraki, C. Trevisan, N. Wardrop, P. Dorny and S. Gabriël (2017); *Taenia solium* in Europe: Still endemic?; *Acta Tropica* 165:96–99

Djordjevic, M., M. Bacic, M. Petricevic, K. Cuperlovic, A. Malakauskas, C.M. Kapel and K.D. Murrell (2003); Social, political and economic factors responsible for the re- emergence of tricinellosis in Serbia: A case study; *Journal of Parasitology* 89(2):226–231

Dorny, P., F. Vercammen, J. Brandt, W. Vansteenkiste, D. Berkvens and S. Geerts (2000); Sero-epidemiological study of *Taenia saginata* cysticercosis in Belgian cattle; *Veterinary Parasitology* 88:43–49

Dorny, P., I. Vallée, L. Alban, J. Boes, P. Boireau, F. Boué, M. Claes, A. Cook, H. Enemar, J. van der Giessen, K. Hunt, M. Howell, M. Kirjušina, K. Nöckler, E. Pozio, P. Rossi, L. Snow, M. Taylor, G. Theodoropoulos, M. Vieira-Pinto and I-A. Zimmer (2010); Development of harmonised schemes for the monitoring and reporting of Cysticercus in animals and foodstuffs in the European Union http://www.efsa.europa.eu/sites/default/files/scientific_output/files/main_documents/34e.pdf accessed November 18 2017

Dupuy, C., C. Morlot, E. Gilot-Fromont, M. Mas, C. Grandmontagne, P. Gilli-Dunoyer, E. Gay and M-P. Callait-Cardinal (2014); Prevalence of *Taenia saginata* cysticercosis in French cattle in 2010; *Veterinary Parasitology* 203:65–72

EC (2000); Opinion of the Scientific Committee on veterinary measure relating to public health on the revision of meat inspection proedures; https://ec.europa.eu/food/sites/food/files/safety/docs/sci-com_scv_out30_en.pdf

ECDC (2010); Surveillance report; https://ecdc.europa.eu/sites/portal/files/media/en/publications/Publications/1011_SUR_Annual_Epidemiological_Report_on_Communicable_Diseases_in_Europe.pdf accessed March 15, 2018

ECDC (2012); Surveillance report, http://ecdc.europa.eu/en/publications/Publications/EU-summary-report-zoonoses-food-borne-outbreaks-2012.pdf accessed April 2016

ECDC (2013); Surveillance report, EFSA Journal 2013;11(4):3129 https://ecdc.europa.eu/sites/portal/files/media/en/publications/Publications/zoonoses-food-outbreaks-report-2011-ecdc-efsa.pdf accessed March 29,2018

ECDC (2014); Surveillance report EFSA Journal 2014;12(2):3547 https://ecdc.europa.eu/sites/portal/files/media/en/publications/Publications/EU-summary-report-zoonoses-food-borne-outbreaks-2012.pdf accessed March 29 2018

ECDC (2015a); Surveillance report; EFSA Journal 2015;13(1):3991 https://ecdc.europa.eu/sites/portal/files/media/en/publications/Publications/EU-summary-report-trends-sources-zoonoses-2013.pdf accessed March 29 2018

ECDC (2015b); The European Union summary report on trends and sources of zoonoses, zoonotic agents and food-borne outbreaks in 2014; EFSA Journal 2015;13(12):4329 https://ecdc.europa.eu/sites/portal/files/media/en/publications/Publications/zoonoses-trends-sources-EU-summary-report-2014.pdf accessed March 29 2018

EFSA (2000); Scientific opinion on veterinary measures relating to public health on the control of taeniosis/cycsticercosis in man and animals; https://ec.europa.eu/food/sites/food/files/safety/docs/sci-com_scv_out36_en.pdf accessed November 18 2017

EFSA (2011); Scientific opinion on the public health hazards to be covered by inspection of meat (swine); *EFSA Journal 2011* 9(10):2351 http://onlinelibrary.wiley.com/doi/10.2903/j.efsa.2011.2351/epdf

EFSA (2015); The European Union summary report on trends and sources of zoonoses, zoonotic agents and food-borne outbreaks in 2013; Scientific Report Of EFSA and ECDC; *EFSA Journal* 13(1):3991

Elkhtam, A.O., I.A. Mostafa and R.R. Shawish (2016); Prevalence and economic impact of cysticercus bovis in slaughtered cattle in Menofia Province, Egypt; Alexandria *Journal of Veterinary Sciences* 50(1):130–134

Fabiani, S. and F. Bruschi (2013); Neurocysticercosis in Europe: Still a public health concern not only for imported cases; *Acta Tropica* 128:18–26

Faber, M., S. Schink, A. Mayer-Scholl, C. Ziesch, R. Schönfelder, H. Wichmann-Schauer, K. Stark, and K. Nöckler (2015); Outbreak of trichinellosis due to wild boar meat and evaluation of the effectiveness of post exposure prophylaxis, Germany 2013; *Clinical Infectious Diseases* 60(12):98–104

Featherstone, C., R. Reichel and S. Mitchell (n.d.); Cysticercus bovis infection in fattened cattle from several farms in the same locality in England; APHA http://ahvla.defra.gov.uk/documents/surveillance/diseases/para-cbovis-cases-poster.pdf accessed November 16 2017

Food Standards Agency (2009); Food Handlers: Fitness to Work https://www.food.gov.uk/sites/default/files/multimedia/pdfs/publication/fitnesstoworkguide09v3.pdf

Gabriël, S., M.V. Johansen, E. Pozio, G.S.A. Smit, B. Devleesschauwer, A. Allepuz, E. Papadopoulos, J. van der Giessen and P. Dorny (2013); Human migration and pig/pork import in the European Union: What are the implications for *Taenia solium* infections? *Veterinary Parasitology* 213:38–45

Garcia, H., A. Gonzalez, C. Evans and R. Gilman (2003); *Taenia solium* cysticercosis; *Lancet* 362(9383):547–556

Gilman R.H., A.E. Gonzalez, F. Llanos-Zavalaga, V.C.W. Tsang, H.H. Garcia for The Cysticercosis Working Group in Peru (2012); Prevention and control of *Taenia solium* taeniasis/cysticercosis in Peru; *Pathogens and Global Health* 106(5):312–318

Gomez-Garcia, V., J. Hernandez-Quero and M. Rodriguez-Osorio (2003); Human infection with *trichinella britovi* in Granada, Spain; *The American Journal of Tropical Medicine and Hygiene* 68(4):463–464

Gracey, J.F. (1981); Thornton's Meat Hygiene, 7th edition; Balliere Tindall; London

Hill, A., A. Brouwer, N. Donaldson, S. Lambton, S. Buncic and I. Griffiths (2013); A risk and benefit assessment for visual-only meat inspection of indoor and outdoor pigs in the United Kingdom; *Food Control* 30:255–264

Hill, A., V. Horigan, K. Clarke, T. Dewé, K. Stärk, S.O'Brien and S. Buncic (2014); A qualitative risk assessment for visual-only post-mortem meat inspection of cattle, sheep, goats and farmed/wild deer; *Food Control* 38(2014):96–103

Hira, P., I. Francis, N.A. Abdella, R. Gupta, F.M. Al-Ali, S. Grover, N. Khalid, S. Abdeen, J. Iqbal, M. Wilson and V. Tsang (2004); Cysticercosis: Imported and autochthonous infections in Kuwait; *Transactions of the Royal Society of Tropical Medicine and Hygiene* 98:233–239

Hoberg, E. (2002); *Taenia* tapeworms: Their biology, evolution and socioeconomic significance; *Microbes and Infection* 4:859–866

Kelley, J., T. Elliott, T. Beddoe, G. Anderson, P. Skuce, and T. Spithill (2016); Current threat of Triclabendazole resistance in *Fasciola hepatica*; *Trends in Parasitology* 32(6):458–469

Kenyon, F., N.D. Sargison, P.J. Skuce and F. Jackson (2009); Sheep helminth parasitic disease in south eastern Scotland arising as a possible consequence of climate change; *Veterinary Parasitology* 163:293–297

Kern, P., K. Bardonnet, E. Renner, H. Auer, Z. Pawlowski, R.W. Ammann, D.A. Vuitton and the European Echinococcosis Registry (2003); European Echinococcosis Registry: Human Alveolar Echinococcosis, Europe, 1982–2000; *Emerging Infectious Diseases* 9(3):343–349

Khan, F., Y.Z. Imam, H. Kamel and M. Shafaee (2011); Neurocysticercosis in Qatari patients: Case reports; *Travel Medicine and Infectious Disease* 9(6):298–302

Laranjo-González, M., B. Devleesschauwer, C. Trevisan, A. Allepuz, S. Sotiraki, A. Abraham, M. Boaventura Afonso, J. Blocher, L. Cardoso, J. Manuel Correia da Costa, P. Dorny, S. Gabriël, J. Gomes, M. Gómez-Morales, P. Jokelainen, M. Kaminski, B. Krt, P. Magnussen, L. Robertson, V. Schmidt, E. Schmutzhard, G. Smit, B. Šoba, C. Stensvold, J. Starič, K. Troell, A. Vergles Rataj, M. Vieira-Pinto, M. Vilhena, N. Wardrop, A. Winkler and V. Dermauw (2017); Epidemiology of taeniosis/cysticercosis in Europe, a systematic review: Western Europe; *Parasites and Vectors* 10:349

Liu, M. and P. Boireau (2002); Trichinellosis in China: Epidemiology and control; *Trends in Parasitology* 18(12):553–556

Marshall, L., B.C. Prakashbabu, J.P. Ferreira, K. Staerk and J. Guitian (2015); Potential use of farm of origin information for more targeted inspection of Cysticercus bovis (FS517002); RVC, University of London; https://www.food.gov.uk/sites/default/files/fs517002finalreport.pdf accessed November 16 2017

Mazeri, S., G. Rydevik, I. Handel, M. Bronsvoort and N. Sargison (2017); Estimation of the impact of *Fasciola hepatica* infection on time taken for UK beef cattle to reach slaughter weight; *Nature Scientific Reports* 7:7319 DOI: 10.1038/s41598-017-07396-1

Meštrović, T., M. Sviben, T. Vilibić-Čavlek, S. Ljubin-Sternak, I. Tabain, and G. Mlinarić-Galinović (2012); Seroprevalence of *Taenia solium* infections in Croatian patients presenting with epilepsy; *Journal of Helminthology* 86(3):259–262

Nelson, M., T.L. Wright, A. Pierce and R.A. Krogwald (2003); A common source outbreak of trichinosis from consumption of bear meat; *Journal of Environmental Health* 65(9):16–19

O'Keefe, K., M.L. Eberhard, S.C. Shafir, P. Wilkins, L.R. Ash and F.J. Sorvillo (2015); Cysticercosis-related hospitalizations in the United States, 1998–2011; *American Journal of Tropical Medicine and Hygiene* 92(2):354–359

O'Neal, S.E., L.M. Moyano, V. Ayvar, S. Rodriguez, C. Gavidia, P. Wilkins, R. Gilman, H. Garcia and A. Gonzalez, for The Cysticercosis Working Group in Peru (2014); Ring-screening to control endemic transmission of *Taenia solium*; *PLOS Neglected Tropical Diseases* 8(9):e3125 https://doi.org/10.1371/journal.pntd.0003125

Raether, W. and H. Hanel (2003); Epidemiology, clinical manifestations and diagnosis of zoonotic cestode infections: An update; *Parasitology Research* 91:412–438

Regulation (EC) No 854/2004 Official controls on the products of animal origin intended for human consumption; OJ L139/2004

Rondelaud,D., P. Vignoles, M. Arbrous and G. Dreyfuss (2001); The definitive and inter-mediate hosts of *Fasciola hepatica* in the natural watercress beds in central France; *Parasitology Research* 87:475–478

Rondelaud, D., G. Dreyfuss, B. Bouteil and M. Dardé (2000); Changes in human fascio-lois in a temperate area: About some observations in a 28 year period in central France; *Parasitology Research* 86:753–787

Schantz, P.M., A. Moore, J. Munoz, B. Hartman, J.A. Schaefer, A.M. Aron, D. Persaud, E. Sarti, M. Wilson and A. Flisser (1992); Neurocysticercosis in an Orthodox Jewish com-munity in New York City; *New England Journal of Medicine* 327:692–695.

Tembo, A. and P. Craig (2015); *Taenia saginata* taeniosis: Copro-antigen time-course in a voluntary self-infection; *Journal of Helminthology* 89(5):612–619

Thorslund, C., M. Aaslyng and J. Lassen (2017); Perceived importance and responsibility for market-driven pig welfare: Literature review; *Meat Science* 125:37–45

Wang, Z., X. Wang and X. Liu (2008); Echinococcosis in China, a Review of the Epidemi-ology of *Echinococcus* spp.; *EcoHealth* 5:115–126

WHO   (2008);   http://www.who.int/zoonoses/diseases/echinococcosis/en/index.html accessed November 18 2017

WHO (2017); Taeniasis/cysticercosis fact sheet http://www.who.int/mediacentre/factsheets/fs376/en/ accessed November 18 2017

Wilson, A. (1998); *Wilson's Practical Meat Inspection*, 6th edition; ed. Wilson W.G; Black-well Science 2001

Zammarchi, L., M. Strohmeyer, F. Bartalesi, E. Bruno, J. Muñoz and D. Buonfrate, The COHEMI Project Study Group (2013); Epidemiology and Management of Cysticer-cosis and *Taenia solium* Taeniasis in Europe, Systematic Review 1990–2011; *PLoS ONE* 8(7):e69537 http://doi.org/10.1371/journal.pone.0069537 accessed November 18 2017

7 Food fraud

The previous chapters have focused on food safety risks. The topic in this chapter, food fraud, is bigger than just safety. Food fraud occurs when the integrity of food is deliberately compromised in some way. The food *may* be rendered unsafe but not always. It can still be fit to eat but not of the nature, substance or quality required. The characteristics of food fraud are that it is:

- intentional
- carried out for economic gain
- concealed

The intentional nature of the compromise and its concealment means that the traditional approaches to food control have limited value. Food inspection is generally aimed at identifying hazards that arise through poor understanding or accidental contamination. Most food business operators would prefer not to sell their customers contaminated food and the legislation reflects that principle. In the UK, non-compliance with food safety legislation is a criminal offence, but it is a regulatory offence, designed to protect the public from inadvertent contamination. Food fraud is also considered a crime, but the deliberate nature of the action makes it, in many cases, morally more unacceptable, even if there is no public health risk. In his review on the integrity and assurance of food supply networks (Elliott 2014), Professor Elliott considers that when food fraud becomes an organised activity it should be defined as 'food crime'. There is evidence that sectors of the food industry have been targeted by organised criminal gangs who are committing offences such as theft, misrepresentation, sale of illegal products and money laundering (van Uhm and Siegel 2016, HM Revenue and Customs 2017). As a consequence, it is important that additional specialist support is available for enforcement officers whose training, powers and procedures are aimed at detecting and controlling accidental regulatory non-compliance rather than organised crime. To that end the Food Standards Agency has established a National Food Crime Unit in the UK whose first task has been to establish a baseline understanding of the extent of food crime in Denmark, Italy, Germany and the Netherlands, which all have long established units with specialist expertise to deal with food crime. However, comforting as it may be to blame rogue outsiders, there is also evidence that systematic fraud is occurring within the industry, sanctioned or tolerated by the business. In this respect, food fraud resembles the professional or 'white collar' crime described by Dellaportas (2013) where accountants used their specialist technical knowledge and privileged position of trust to defraud clients and employers.

Vulnerability

The food industry is open to fraud for two reasons. The first is because, in the modern world, most consumers acquire food as the result of a series of commercial transactions. The food industry, as would be expected in any manufacturing or retail based sector, aims to make a profit from the process. Because it is a large and vibrant industry, the sums involved can be significant. While the vast majority of the food industry is comprised of honest and honourable businesses, the opportunity to make money illegally will also present itself to the criminally minded, as in any other commercial sector. The food industry is based on a complex, global supply chain which separates consumers from producers. This is the second aspect which provides potential for fraudulent transactions. There are typically many steps between the primary producer and final sale. At each of these, the food is likely to be processed, packaged, combined or otherwise changed in such a way that the purchaser is unable to easily evaluate the composition or quality. This provides the opportunity for fraud since the chance that any alteration will be identified is minimised.

Where such an alteration will maximise profit and the fraudster believes that no consequence will result from the alteration, a vulnerability in the food supply is created. The scenario derives from the study of criminology (routine activity theory) (Pustjens *et al.* 2016, van Ruth *et al.* 2017) which suggests that a crime will occur when motivated persons are presented with a suitable target in the absence of controls. The concept of a fraud triangle is similar and uses opportunity, motivation and rationalisation as its three elements. Where a person has the opportunity to commit an illegal act, the motivation to do so and can rationalise the action, fraud will take place. In the fraud triangle, a lack of controls will contribute to the 'opportunity' element (Dellaportas, 2013, Lokanan 2015). Both theories serve as good frameworks to examine the circumstances surrounding food fraud.

Opportunity

Specialist knowledge

Like other manufacturing industries, food production relies heavily on engineering technology and expert staff. This specialist knowledge can help food business operators identify opportunities for fraud that would not be evident to outsiders. With regard to food safety, many of the common contaminants have been researched and characterised. This makes identification and control possible, if not always completely successful. Of course this does not apply to fraud where the choice of contaminant, adulterant or substitute is whatever the food business operator can imagine, access and implement. The combination of specialist knowledge with regard to process and control is demonstrated in the melamine contamination incident in China (Chan *et al.* 2008). The food producer combined understanding of the analysis process (testing for nitrogen as an indicator of protein) with knowledge of the chemical composition of melamine ($C_3H_6N_6$) and its properties to invent a way of stretching the volume of milk which would be undetected through analytical or organoleptic tests. By adding a cheap chemical, the milk was made more profitable. Another example of specialist knowledge (microbiological and chemical) was demonstrated, again with milk, in Brazil. Here the aim appears to have been to cover high bacterial counts and extend the shelf life by reducing spoilage bacteria. Producers added hydrogen peroxide (H_2O_2) to the milk to reduce the bacterial load and then, because this caused a change in pH, demonstrated further their understanding of chemistry by adding acidity regulators (Cardoso *et al.* 2012). Presumably all these chemicals were much cheaper than buying the refrigerated tankers which would have controlled the microbial growth legally. In his report on accounting fraud, Dellaportas (2013) suggested that opportunity, particularly when created by specialist technical knowledge and trust, was the most important of the three aspects in the fraud triangle. There is no doubt that this is relevant to food fraud. The serious frauds referred to previously, and the contamination of beef products with horse (O'Mahony 2013), relied, for their success, on critical knowledge of the process and product as well as the trust between supplier and purchaser.

Weak bonds, lax controls

A factor in the decision to act fraudulently is the likelihood of discovery. If the food can be compromised in a way that is difficult or expensive to detect, an opportunity is created. This will be exacerbated in situations where there are lax controls (industry or government) which allow non-compliance to be ignored or tolerated. Poor cultural norms in a company or sector provide a situation conducive to fraud. Unchecked actions such as bullying or victimisation and bad practices (process and management) will create an environment in which illicit behaviour can flourish (van Ruth *et al.* 2017, Dellaportas 2013). Lokanan (2015) states that the opportunity for fraud, and presumably the likelihood, 'increases as the firm's control structure weakens'. This suggests that chaotic companies with poor procedures or poor adherence to procedures are more vulnerable to fraud. The existence of previous offences or offences in other areas is also considered to be an indicator of a high risk for fraud (van Ruth *et al.* 2017, BOD 2007, FSA 2016a). Companies with a history of non-compliance are likely to normalise the attitude in all areas.

Individual food businesses can demonstrate weak controls which create fraud in an otherwise compliant sector. However, the more general standards and norms in a country can also predispose a sector or product to compromise. Where there is endemic corruption, the dishonesty and lack of transparency tends to create a similar environment in the country's food industry, increasing the risk of fraud. Transparency International ranks 176 countries on an annual basis according to perceived levels of corruption (Anonymous 2016). Countries with a score indicating high levels of corruption, that is, a low numeric score (0 = extremely corrupt, 100 = no corruption at all), also tend to feature significantly in alerts for food crime, for example, Sudan dye contamination of spices (FSA 2015b) and oil (FSA 2015a), supply of bush meat (Chaber *et al.* 2010) and laundering of honey (Everstine *et al.* 2013).

Motivation

The motivation to commit fraud is enhanced economic gain. The universality of the food industry ensures there is great potential. Everyone eats, thereby creating, potentially, seven and a half billion opportunities each day for food to change hands. Only a very small proportion of these exchanges need to be fraudulent for it to be worthwhile from a fraudster's viewpoint, and often only a very small economic advantage to each transaction is needed to result in significant gain, given the large scale of the industry. The motivation to act fraudulently can result from incentive or from pressure.

The food industry is based on primary production. This in turn is affected by natural conditions. Global sourcing, which is such a feature of the modern food industry, does enhance the security of supply by spreading sourcing risk but cannot eliminate all variation in availability for all products. Natural events, extremes of weather and political factors can all reduce supply, temporarily or permanently. When the demand for a product exceeds its supply, its cost will increase. This simple fact can create the pressure to adulterate, dilute or substitute a foodstuff in order to keep production going, or to maintain profitability (Manning and Soon 2014).

Even without critical events such as failed harvests, there can be significant pressure within the food industry which can encourage fraud. Competitive pricing and contracts with stringent penalties ensure the public in the UK have access to an unparalleled variety and quantity of affordable food but there comes a point where it is impossible to reduce the cost of producing a particular food any further. If there continues to be pressure exerted by the purchaser to reduce the price, the producer will either go out of business or be forced to alter the product so it is cheaper to produce (Manning and Soon 2014, van Ruth *et al.* 2017). If the second route is chosen, the main options are to use cheaper ingredients – usually substandard, illegal or alternate materials, or to 'stretch' the production by diluting or bulking. Financial strain of this type is an acknowledged motivator to commit fraud in other sectors (Dellaportas 2013, Lokanan 2015).

Rationalisation

The third point of the fraud triangle is rationalisation. In spite of the commercial nature of the industry and the many opportunities to commit food fraud, the majority of people in the food sector do not appear to do so. According to the fraud triangle theory, in addition to the opportunity and motivation, fraudsters must also be able to rationalise their illegal action. According to Dellaportas (2013), rationalisation can be divided into three routes:

1   Denial of responsibility (e.g. it was the fault of the customer (retailer) who would only renew the contract at a lower price)
2   Denial of injury (e.g. the adulterant will not harm anyone)
3   Denial of victim (e.g. the ultimate consumer is unknown /faceless)

A long and complex food chain not only provides more steps, each with the potential for compromise, but also serves to disconnect producers and consumers, making the denial of victim much easier. The three aspects of the fraud triangle may not apply equally to the decision to commit fraud. In a given circumstance one could be more important than the other two, but all should be present for the illegal activity to occur.

Categories of Food Fraud

It can be helpful to try and categorise the types of fraud to which the food chain is vulnerable. As these are artificial categories, there is some overlap. It is not useful to argue whether something is adulteration or substitution, simulation or misrepresentation. The point of categorising is to assist in identifying some of the ways fraud can be perpetrated. If an example fits into two (or even more) categories, that probably means it is an important issue and needs attention.

1   Adulteration

Adulteration usually refers to the addition of an unacknowledged ingredient to a food. Typically it would make the food cheaper to produce, make an unfit product appear fit for consumption or make a poor quality product appear more desirable so as to command a higher price. The literature abounds with examples of adulteration including the two milk cases mentioned previously (Chan *et al.* 2008, Cardoso *et al.* 2012). Water can also be used fraudulently. The use of excess overglaze in fish to make the product heavier (Vanhaecke *et al.* 2010) or water added to poultry for the same reason could be considered adulteration. Watering down a liquid to extend volume may also need other adulterants added in order to pass analysis as demonstrated by Sanlu in the melamine and milk fraud case (Chan *et al.* 2008). Another example of adulteration is the addition of Sudan dyes (illegal in foods) to enhance the colour of palm oil (FSA 2015a) and spices (FSA 2015b, Genualdi *et al.* 2016, Petrakis *et al.* 2017). Because of the milling and grinding that takes place during production, spices can be very vulnerable to adulteration. In addition to illegal Sudan dyes to improve colour, saffron can be adulterated with various plant materials such as calendula (marigold), safflower and turmeric (Petrakis

and Polissiou 2017). Dried herbs also undergo a process which makes it difficult to identify the contents and have been found to be adulterated. Sampling
of Oregano carried out in the UK found 24% of the samples were adulterated,
most commonly with olive or myrtle leaves (Black *et al.* 2016).

2   Substitution

Closely related to adulteration is substitution. Substitution is where an infe-
rior product is sold in place of the more expensive item. It can also be a form
of adulteration when a cheaper or alternate product is used to bulk out a foodstuff by replacing part of the more valuable ingredient. The contamination of
UK beef products with horse meat is a widely reported example (O'Mahony
2013, Walker *et al.* 2013). It was largely responsible for the commission of
the Elliott Review and the increased focus on fraud in the UK food industry.
Honey is another vulnerable product. Legally, honey should have nothing
added to it (see schedule 1 of The Honey (England) Regulations 2015). However, there are reports where honey has been found to contain high fructose
corn syrup, glucose or other sugar syrups made from beet or cane (Tosun
2013). The fact that many foods are sold as composite products such as pies,
casseroles, puddings and sauces means that, in the final product, it is often
impossible to identify the ingredients without scientific analysis. Substitution
during manufacture with a cheaper raw material such as whiting (*Merlan-
gius merlangus*) for a more expensive material such as cod *(Gadus morhua)*
or haddock (*Melanogrammus aeglefinus*) is unlikely to be detected by the
retailer or final consumer using visual or organoleptic means. The retail price
differential of approximately £5 per kg at time of writing indicates the saving which could be made by replacing some of the cod in a fish product with
the cheaper whiting. Surveys in Canada reveal substitution of lower priced
fish for more expensive species occurring in restaurants and at retail (Oceana
2017, Wong and Hanner 2008).

3   Counterfeiting and simulation

Alcoholic beverages demonstrate the potential for both the options in this
category of fraud. Counterfeiting is where fraudsters pass off a fake product
as a genuine brand. The counterfeit product may actually be in genuine packaging which has been stolen by the criminals. An example was reported by
HM Revenue and Customs (2017). A bottling factory was discovered making
vodka which purported to be No 01 Imperial Vodka Blue. The factory had
bottles with counterfeit labels, and officers seized 1,965 litres of product. By
manufacturing illicitly, the fraudsters avoided paying an estimated £45,000 in
tax on the product. Two years earlier HMRC had identified a similar establishment in Cheshire, producing the same counterfeit vodka. The National Food
Crime Unit (FSA 2016a) considers spirits to be an area of serious concern
with regard to fraud and food crime. The fraudsters avoid paying taxes so

they can undercut the legitimate companies. Also, they are making the drink in uncontrolled conditions which can result in the production of highly toxic fluids. Examples have been reported with high methanol content (Mckee *et al.* 2012) or adulterated with propanol (Newton 2015).

Simulation or 'passing off' is where a product is made to copy or resemble a well-known brand but is produced legitimately. The simulation may copy packaging or shape but is in fact a different product. An example is Vodkat – an alcoholic drink made by Intercontinental Brands, which was a mix of vodka and other alcohols, and looked very similar in style to Smirnoff Vodka. Vodkat was considerably cheaper than Smirnoff Vodka, mainly because it had a lower alcohol content which resulted in lower tax (Stone and Heard 2010). Diageo, the company that owns Smirnoff Vodka initiated a lengthy court case against Intercontinental Brands who have now renamed their product V-Kat Schnapps.

4   Misrepresentation

Misrepresentation is a large and potentially lucrative category. There are a number of products where the consumer is prepared to pay a premium for a characteristic which cannot be confirmed at the point of sale. Examples include organic produce, free range eggs, halal meat and line caught fish. The authenticity of such products cannot be tested – there are no analytical techniques which can distinguish organic raspberries from raspberries that are not grown organically. The same applies to halal slaughter of meat. Halal certification is carried out by a halal certification body (HCB), but there is no test which distinguishes halal slaughtered meat from non-halal. In all cases there is reliance on certification and trust in the supply chain. The inherent limitation is that accreditation schemes evaluate the management of the process rather the specification of the product itself. Certification cannot verify that a product is authentic in the absence of independent tests. In fact it can create a sector in which fraud is more likely as the purchasers are relying on/trusting certification which can be falsified. The increased demand for halal meat in the UK has resulted in a number of cases where non-halal meat was sold as halal (Fuseini *et al.* 2017), although typically these were discovered as a result of contamination with undeclared species. Subsequent investigation into traceability established the lack of authentic certification as well as adulteration.

Products with special or protected designation can also be at risk of misrepresentation. Under Council Regulation 1151/2012 the EU recognises three categories of quality which producers can apply to use:

* Protected designation of origin (PDO). This can apply where all aspects of the production occur in the region. Products with PDO status include Kalamata olive oil, Jersey potatoes, Stilton cheese, Prosciutto di Parma and Parmigiano Reggiano.

- Protected Geographical Indication (PGI) can apply where there is a strong geographical link to a place, region or area but not all the production takes place there – for example some ingredients may come from outside the region. Cornish pasties have PGI status, as do Melton Mowbray pies.
- Traditional speciality guaranteed (TSG) is a mark which reflects traditional production methods or composition. Traditionally farmed Gloucestershire Old Spots pork and Bramley apple pie filling are examples of a products with TSG status.

Producers can apply to the European Commission for protection of their product based on one of these categories. The application is assessed and, if protection is awarded, the producer is required to submit to third party certification on a regular basis.

Products with special or protected designation usually command a price premium or competitive advantage over non-designated products. This offers an opportunity for fraudsters to misrepresent products which appear similar to the special product but which are not compliant. For some foods there are analytical techniques which can help establish origin, for example trace-element composition and stable-isotope ratio can evaluate the origins of dairy products, oils, coffee, tea, honey and a number of other products (Gonzalvez *et al.* 2009, Grundy *et al.* 2012), meaning that these can be sampled and tested to verify authenticity.

Foods with limited supply can be at significant risk from fraud. In circumstances where there is a poor harvest but steady demand, producers can be tempted to temporarily adulterate or substitute to meet existing contracts. Difficulty in meeting expectation also applies when consumer demand increases but where supply is limited or requires a long lead in. Manuka honey is an example of a product where both issues apply, creating opportunities for a variety of types of fraud, including at least, adulteration, misrepresentation, counterfeit and simulation. Manuka honey is a monofloral honey produced from a particular plant, the New Zealand Myrtle (*Leptospermum scoparium*), which grows only in certain parts of New Zealand and Australia. This honey has anti-bacterial properties which have been shown to be effective against a number of pathogenic species (Allen *et al.* 1991) including methicillin-resistant *S. aureus* (MRSA) (Lin *et al.* 2017). The honey is used medicinally in hospitals but is also in demand by the public after comments in the popular press and endorsements by celebrities suggesting it can confer a variety of health benefits. Producing more to meet the increasing demand is not a quick or easy option. Seedlings of the New Zealand Myrtle take 8–13 years from planting to produce substantial quantities of nectar, even under ideal growing conditions (MacIntyre 2017) and then the bees need to be encouraged to use it (apparently they prefer clover). It is difficult to establish exactly how much Manuka honey is produced but according the Ministry for Primary Industries (MPI), the entire honey production of New Zealand is only 15,000–20,000 tonnes per annum. A small part of this is Manuka. According to the Elliott review, 1700 tonnes of Manuka honey are produced annually in New Zealand while 1800 tonnes appear to be sold each year in the UK (Elliott 2014)[1]. The inevitable conclusion is that a great deal of the product sold globally as Manuka honey must be fraudulent. The FSA 2014–2015 sampling programme included Manuka honey, and 34% of the samples tested were found to be unsatisfactory (FSA 2016b). To protect this valuable commodity, in December 2017, the MPI were able to establish a definition and testing requirement for Manuka honey which will now apply to all exports from New Zealand (MPI 2017). This new requirement should help to reduce the sale of fraudulent Manuka honey in the future.

5   Illegal products

Products can be illegal for a number of reasons. They can fail to reach regulatory standards, such as animal by-products which are sold for human consumption. They can also be illegal if they are produced in an unregulated country. For example, products of animal origin (POA) which are to be imported into an EU member state must originate from a country which has been approved to export that product to the EU. A country can be approved to export some products of animal origin but not others – such as Iran. Iran is approved for the export of fisheries products and treated stomachs, bladders and intestines (sections VIII and XIII of Regulation EC 853/2004) but not for any other POA. Therefore, it is possible to import caviar legally from Iran but not tins of kalleh paacheh (casserole of sheep brain and feet) or other meat products. Some high risk products not of animal origin (PNOAO) can also attract additional controls, occasionally being banned from import. An example would include the prohibition on import of dried beans from Nigeria due to high levels of the pesticide dichlorvos under Commission Regulation (EU) 2016/874 or the ban on import of honey from China under Commission Decision 2002/994/EC, now lifted (Wei *et al.* 2012). Fraud occurs when products from an unapproved or prohibited country are trans-shipped through an approved country and then into the EU. The National Food Crime Unit mentions this process with regard to banned products from India being transited through the UAE, thereby hiding the true origin. This process is often referred to as 'laundering'. Honey laundering is a well-documented issue in the US (Everstine *et al.* 2013) with various treatments occurring, such as filtering out of the pollen, in an attempt to hide the true origin.

Another possibility for food crime is when food is produced illegally – for example, the production of smokies. Regulation (EC) No 853/2004 annex III, section I chapter IV (8) requires that carcasses of ungulates (except pigs) destined for human consumption are skinned after slaughter.

Smokies are produced by leaving the skin on the slaughtered sheep and burning off the wool. This produces a yellow appearance on the carcass and imparts a smoky flavour to the meat. It is a traditional delicacy in West Africa and in UK cities such as London with residents of African origin. There is no particular health risk associated with production of smokies, but leaving the skin on means it is illegal to place the product on the market in the EU. The FSA (2010) conducted research into the health implications and found there was no reason (apart from the fact it contravened EU law) that smokies could not be produced hygienically. The Agency approached the EC with a view to altering Regulation (EC) No 853/2004, but so far there does not appear to be any amendment which permits production of smokies. Because there is high demand for the product and no legal way of meeting this demand, the opportunity is being exploited by criminal gangs (Anonymous 2014a). There can be multiple problems associated with the illegal slaughter of meat. Uninspected sheep may still have Specified Risk Material (SRM) attached, creating a potential health risk to the consumers, and they are likely to have been slaughtered, dressed and transported in unhygienic conditions with no temperature control. There also appear to be animal welfare issues, waste (animal by-products) disposal problems and sheep rustling associated with the uncontrolled production (FSA 2016a).

An illegal product with an international dimension is bush meat. Bush meat is wild meat, typically sourced from Africa, and smuggled into the EU. It can comprise animals which are not approved for human consumption in Europe, many of which are endangered (Bowen-Jones and Pendry, 1999) and none of which will have been inspected. Chaber *et al.* (2010) checked 29 flights (40% of the total) from West and Central African countries landing in Paris during a single week and found 7% of those searched were carrying bush meat. Based on this sample they estimate that approximately 273 tonnes of bush meat enters the EU annually through Roissy-Charles de Gaulle airport. Trade in 39% of the species identified was either banned or restricted under the Convention on International Trade in Endangered Species of Wild Fauna and Flora (CITES).

Poaching can also be an issue for other endangered species such as the sturgeon. Cohen (1997) reports on an American poaching ring that, over a five year period, targeted the white sturgeon, *Acipenser transmontanus*, in the lower Columbia River in Washington State. The roe was being sent to the Hansen Caviar Company in New Jersey. There was a double fraud in this case. Not only was the caviar illegal, as *Acipenser transmontanus* is a protected species and cannot be legally harvested, but some of the roe was being re-labelled as imported beluga or osetra caviar before being sold At the time, the price differential between American caviar and imported beluga was estimated to be over $500 per pound, making it a very lucrative fraud. Experts estimated that the ring had supplied over 3,000 pounds of caviar with the destruction of approximately 2,000 fish.

At risk foods

Identifying food fraud can be challenging. Given the size and complexity of the food industry and the opportunities at every step, it is important to try and identify any processes or types of foods which may be at risk. Table 7.1 summarises some of the characteristics which could make foods vulnerable to fraud. These include:

1   **Common foods** that everyone eats. A large sales volume means that a small saving per item can result in a substantial increase in profit.
2   **Expensive or luxury foods.** This is the opposite of common foods – product with a large price per unit only needs a small increase in quantity to ensure a substantial increase in profit.
3   **Products with special significance.** Where these are important to a particular group of consumers it allows careful targeting of the fraudulent product and exploitation of the group.
4   **Rapidly emerging trend, limited source.** Products that suddenly become fashionable can be vulnerable when the supply is limited. A sudden increase in the demand for a product like pomegranate juice, for example, where there are limited existing supplies in inaccessible places and new trees require 3–6 years to produce fruit (USAID 2008), is likely to be open to fraud. Celebrity endorsement of fresh kale juice, on the other hand, would not pose such a challenge for the industry because kale is an annual vegetable that grows very easily in Northern Europe and needs only a few months to mature.
5   **Steady demand, reduced supply.** When normal supply of a product is interrupted through natural disaster, poor harvest or political instability but the demand remains the same, vulnerability can be created. In the autumn/winter of 2017 wildfires impacted heavily on the wine growing regions of California (Napa Valley, Sonoma County and other important production areas). Reports suggest the damage was limited for the 2017 vintage but evaluating the impact on future production must wait until the winter pruning and 2018 growth (Worobiec 2017). Limited supply in future years could create a potential vulnerability.

Controls

The control of food fraud and food crime cannot be left to the enforcement authorities. It must be a four way partnership involving the enforcement authorities, the food industry, national agencies and the consumer. The food industry needs to take a lead in the control of fraud. It is a victim of food crime as well as a perpetrator. Businesses that unknowingly buy compromised food are being exploited and defrauded. If the problem is detected, the business then bears the cost of recall, legal costs if enforcement action results and damage to reputation. Gee *et al.* (2014) state that food fraud impacts on the financial stability of the industry and causes food to be more expensive. They consider 73 food and drink companies listed on the London Stock Exchange and suggest that elimination of food fraud could improve their profitability by £4.48 billion. They estimate that three of the companies would become profitable instead of loss making.

Table 7.1 Examples of vulnerable food types

At risk	Types of fraud	Examples
Common foods Foods where there is a high production volume. A small saving on every item produces large profit.	Adulteration Dilution Bulking with water or other fillers Substitution Illegal supply, laundering Extending shelf life	Milk (Chan *et al.* 2008, Cardoso *et al.* 2012) Meat (O'Mahony 2013, Walker *et al.* 2013) Fish (van Haecke *et al.* 2010, Oceana 2017, Everstine *et al.* 2013 summary, Wong and Hanner 2008) Honey (Tosun 2013, Everstine *et al.* 2013 summary) Oil (Genualdi *et al.* 2016, FSA 2015a, Everstine *et al.* 2013 summary) Juice (Everstine *et al.* 2013 summary, GAO 1995)
Expensive or luxury foods High value products, especially when sourced from countries with weak food control systems or endemic corruption.	Adulteration Substitution Mislabelling Counterfeit Illegal supply	Caviar (Cohen 1997; van Uhm and Siegel 2016) Alcoholic drinks, spirits and wines (Mckee *et al.* 2012, Newton 2015, Stone and Heard 2010, Everstine *et al.* 2013 summary,) Spices e.g. Saffron (Petrakis and Polissiou 2017) Dried herbs e.g. Oregano (Black *et al.* 2016)
Products with special significance These are frequently exploited in a seriously criminal way which shows no respect for the consumers or the product.	Illegal supply Substitution Mislabelling	Smokies (Anonymous 2014a) Bush meat (Chaber *et al.* 2010) Certified products like halal food (Fuseini *et al.* 2017), organic and free-range foods Products with a protected status
Emerging trend Increased demand for products with limited supply and a long lead in time.	Adulteration Substitution Mislabelling Counterfeit Dilution Bulking with water or other fillers	Manuka honey (FSA 2016b; Elliott 2014) Pomegranate juice (Everstine *et al.* 2013 summary)
Steady demand, reduced supply Temporary interruption due to poor harvest, inclement weather, political instability.	Adulteration Substitution Mislabelling Bulking	Potentially California wine (Worobiec 2017)

While there are examples of organised criminal gangs targeting sectors of the industry, the National Fraud Authority (2013) survey indicated that 49% of fraud that occurred in the private sector was 'insider enabled'. If this proportion is applicable to the food industry, it means that the best way forward is to develop controls from within. The role of high standards of compliance, strong management controls, integrity and ethical behaviour in reducing the opportunity for fraud within a company are stressed by a number of experts. Whistle blowing is also an important detection tool in discovering insider fraud (van Ruth *et al.* 2017, Elliott 2014) and should be treated as a potential source. There is a tendency by some inspectors to dismiss insider complaints as a 'disgruntled employee' and not follow up to establish whether there is any substance to the report.

In addition to the general good practices already mentioned, industries need to be proactive and carry out assessments of potential vulnerabilities. To assist food business operators, a number of evaluation tools have been developed and published. Some include assessments for other threats, such as terrorist action. While these tools are aimed at the food industry, they are also useful for food inspectors. Many of the questions and suggestions in the tools can be used during an inspection to evaluate the food business operator's awareness of vulnerability to fraud and how well s/he is controlling the process and raw materials. Five of these tools are listed below.

1   **CARVER + shock (FDA 2009)**

   The CARVER + shock evaluation tool was developed by the U.S. Food and Drug Administration to help food business operators identify vulnerabilities in their companies. It is primarily a food defence tool using terms like 'attack' rather than hazard but it helps a food business operator focus on the weak spots and resilience within the business. If economically motivated adulteration by a supplier was defined as the 'threat', for example, the software could be used in an evaluation of food crime vulnerability. The system is probably best suited to major companies. It is time consuming to use but thorough.

2   **SSAFE Food Fraud Tool (SSAFE 2017)**

   SSAFE is a non-profit organisation with members from major multinational food companies. The organisation has collaborated with Wageningen University and Price Waterhouse Cooper (PWC) to develop an online food fraud vulnerability assessment tool. Food business operators wishing to use the tool register and then complete fifty questions which follow a multiple choice answer format. The format makes it more accessible and much less time consuming than the CARVER + shock. After completion, the food business operator is sent a pdf summary of responses and a spider web diagram relating to opportunities, motivation and control measures. It can be used for most sectors but would probably appeal more to large businesses rather than SMEs. According to the developers, it is designed to support businesses wishing to take part in the Global Food Safety Initiative (GFSI). For a discussion of the parameters used to develop the tool, see van Ruth *et al.* 2017.

3   **TACCP (Anonymous 2014b)**

The FSA, DEFRA and BSI collaborated to produce PAS 96:2014 Guide to protecting and defending food and drink from deliberate attack. This guide (*not* a BSI standard) uses a process similar to HACCP to help food business operators evaluate vulnerabilities in their business. It can be used to assess fraud vulnerability and also for defence if the food business operator wishes. The advantage is that it draws on principles that are already familiar to many food business operators such as flow charts, evaluation of priority (risk) through assessing the impact and likelihood of the event, and development of appropriate controls as needed.

4   **Food Authenticity (FDF n.d.)**

The Food and Drink Federation (FDF) have developed and published a five step plan which helps businesses evaluate vulnerabilities to fraud and consider any changes needed to protect the company. It begins with mapping their supply chain, then identifying issues, assessing risk and planning controls. The fifth step is implementation, including review. The guide uses straightforward questions which food business operators will be able to answer quickly and easily from their knowledge of the business. It does not need any specialist equipment and the language is practical and clear. It gives a framework that focuses on key aspects which could create an opportunity for fraud. It is not sector specific and is appropriate for SMEs.

5   **Guidance on the Authenticity of Herbs and Spices (Anonymous n.d.)**

This guidance is hosted on the FDF website but is the result of collaboration between the FDF, British Retail Consortium (BRC) and Seasoning and Spices Association (SSA). It provides guidance in the form of a decision tree which helps food business operators in the spice and herb sector to identify potential vulnerabilities. There is guidance on control measures, examples of common adulterants and testing methods which can be used to identify or authenticate products, species names and harvest charts, including countries of origin. It is specialist but valuable for a high risk sector.

There are a number of issues that make food fraud and food crime difficult for the food authorities to control. One very significant issue is what might be called the 'wilderness aspect'. Food safety controls are designed to address known hazards which have been characterised and described. With food fraud and food crime, competent authorities are dealing with what Manning and Soon (2014) call 'unknown unknowns'. Only fraudsters know what has been done to the food and they are trying very hard to hide it. So an alteration which was created through specialist knowledge and designed to be undetected needs to be identified by an outsider whose training is to deal with accidental hygiene noncompliance. This is certainly a challenge for inspectors. Probably the way to address it is to continue doing what inspectors do best – ask nosey questions and keep going until the answer makes sense. Presumably Sanlu had to receive deliveries of melamine in order to mix it with their milk and it would have been stored somewhere, measured in something and added somehow to the product. Although if a company went to the extremes exhibited by Sun Up Foods, it might be difficult for even the most diligent inspector to spot. Sun Up Foods were found to be systematically diluting their 'unsweetened' orange juice with 10–20% beet sugar. They built hidden pipework and secret doors into holding tanks, accepted deliveries of the liquid sugar only in the middle of the night and falsified the invoices to list the delivered ingredient as 'orange concentrate' (GAO 1995).

In order to successfully address food fraud and crime, national agencies such as the FSA and National Food Crime unit will need to support local officers with intelligence. Some will come from horizon scanning and international networks, but an essential source of information is the food industry. The challenge is to find a way of sharing the results of sampling and audits in a way which protects the compliant businesses but leaves the fraudsters exposed. That will help target enforcement and delivery of controls where it is most effective.

Note

1 Please note the original reference for this data is no longer available on the MPI webpage.

References

Allen, K., P. Molan and G. Reid (1991); A survey of the antibacterial activity of some New Zealand honeys; *Journal of Pharmacy and Pharmacology* 43(12):817–882

Anonymous (2014a); Food Safety: Croydon destroys smokies; The EHP Jul 22, 2014 https://theehp.com/2014/07/22/food-safety-croydon-destroys-smokies/ accessed November 2017

Anonymous (2014b); PAS 96:2014 Guide to protecting and defending food and drink from deliberate attack https://www.food.gov.uk/sites/default/files/pas96-2014-food-drink-protection-guide.pdf accessed November 2017

Anonymous (2016); Corruptions perception index; Transparency International; https://www.transparency.org/news/feature/corruption_perceptions_index_2016 accessed November 2017

Anonymous (n.d.); Guidance on the Authenticity of Herbs and Spices; Industry best practice on assessing and protecting culinary dried herbs and spices https://www.fdf.org.uk/corporate_pubs/guidance-herbsandspices.pdf accessed November 2017

Black, C., S. Haughey, O. Chevallier, P. Galvin-King and C. Elliott (2016); A comprehensive strategy to detect the fraudulent adulteration of herbs: The oregano approach; *Food Chemistry* 210:551–557

BOD (2007); Focus on Fraud; Special Investigative Platform; Ministry of Social Affairs and Employment, The Hague

Bowen-Jones, E. and S. Pendry (1999);The threat to primates and other mammals from the bushmeat trade in Africa, and how this threat could be diminished; *Oryx* 33:233–246

Cardoso, C.F., A.G. Cruz, U.M. Pinto and J.A.F. Faria (2012); Chapter 33: Investigating the adulteration of UHT milk in Brazil; In: *Case Studies in Food Safety and Authenticity: Lessons from Real-Life Situations*; ed. Jeffrey Hoorfar; Woodhead Publishing

Chaber, A., L. Allebone-Webb, S.Y. Lignereux, A.A. Cunningham and J.M. Rowcliffe (2010), The scale of illegal meat importation from Africa to Europe via Paris; *Conservation Letters* 3:317–321

Chan, E., S.M. Griffiths and C.W. Chan(2008); Public-health risks of melamine in milk products; *Lancet* 372:1444–5

Cohen, A. (1997); Sturgeon poaching and black market caviar: A case study; *Environmental Biology of Fishes* 48:423–426

Dellaportas, S. (2013); Conversations with inmate accountants: Motivation, opportunity and the fraud triangle; *Accounting Forum* 37(1):29–39

Elliott, C. (2014); Elliott Review into the Integrity and Assurance of Food Supply Networks-Final Report; https://www.gov.uk/government/uploads/system/uploads/attachment_data/file/350726/elliot-review-final-report-july2014.pdf accessed December 11, 2017

Everstine, K., J. Spink and S. Kennedy (2013); Economically motivated adulteration (EMA) of food: Common characteristics of EMA incidents; Journal of Food Protection; 76(4):723–735

FDA (2009); CARVER + shock https://www.fda.gov/Food/FoodDefense/FoodDefense Programs/ucm376791.htm accessed December 11, 2017

FDF (n.d.); Food Authenticity https://www.fdf.org.uk/corporate_pubs/Food-Authenticity-guide-2014.pdf accessed December 11, 2017

FSA (2010); Report on research into the production of smoked skin-on sheep meat https://www.food.gov.uk/sites/default/files/multimedia/pdfs/board/fsa100104.pdf accessed December 11, 2017

FSA (2015a); Product recall: Unlabelled Ghanaian palm oil found to contain Sudan IV sold at Kemtoy Miyan Cash & Carry https://www.food.gov.uk/search?keyword=sudan%20 dye& accessed March 15 2018

FSA (2015b); Product recall: Yekta Foods recalls Sommak spice because it contains illegal dyes https://www.food.gov.uk/news-updates/news/2015/13932/yekta-foods-recalls-sommak-spice-illegal-dyes accessed March 15 2018

FSA (2016a); Food Crime Annual Strategic Assessment: A 2016 baseline https://www.food.gov.uk/sites/default/files/fsa-food-crime-assessment-2016.pdf accessed March 15 2018

FSA (2016b); Surveillance activity of Manuka honey on the UK market https://www.food.gov.uk/sites/default/files/manukareport-final-2016.pdf accessed March 15 2018

Fuseini, A., S.B. Wotton, T.G. Knowles and P.J. Hadley (2017); Halal Meat Fraud and Safety Issues in the UK: A review in the Context of the European Union; *Food Ethics* 1(2):127–142.

GAO (1995) Fruit Juice Adulteration; Report to the Congressional Committees; http://www.gao.gov/assets/230/221856.pdf accessed December 11, 2017

Gee, J., L. Jack and M. Button (2014); Minimising fraud and maximising value in the UK food and drink sector; PKF Littlejohn LLP http://www.port.ac.uk/media/contacts-and-departments/icjs/ccfs/PKF_LittleJohn_-_Fraud_in_the_food_sector_report.pdf accessed December 11, 2017

Genualdi S., S. MacMahon, K. Robbins, S. Farris, N. Shyong and L. DeJager (2016); Method development and survey of Sudan I–IV in palm oil and chilli spices in the Washington, DC, area; *Food Additives & Contaminants Part A: Chemistry, analysis, control, exposure & risk assessment* 33(4):583–591 doi:10.1080/19440049.2016.1147986.

Gonzalvez, A., S. Armenta, M. de la Guardia (2009); Trace-element composition and stable-isotope ratio for discrimination of foods with Protected Designation of Origin; *Trends in Analytical Chemistry* 28(11):1295–1311

Grundy, H., S. Kelly, A. Charlton, J. Donarski, S. Hird, H. Hird and M.Collins (2012); Food Authenticity and Food fraud research: Achievements and Emerging Issues; *Journal of the Association of Public Analysts* (online) 40:65–68

HM Revenue & Customs (2017); Fake vodka factory in Liverpool http://www.mynews desk.com/uk/hm-revenue-customs-hmrc/pressreleases/fake-vodka-factory-found-in-liverpool-2076750 accessed December 11, 2017

Lin,B., K.Loomes; G. Prijic; R. Schlothauer and J. Stephens (2017); Lepteridine as a unique fluorescent marker for the authentication of manuka honey; *Food Chemistry* 225:175–180

Lokanan, M. (2015); Challenges to the fraud triangle: Questions on its usefulness; *Accounting Forum* 39(3):201–224

Manning, L. and J.M.Soon (2014); Developing systems to control food adulteration; *Food Policy* 49:23–32

MacIntyre, P. (2017); Progress review of the high performance Manuka plantations primary growth partnership programme, Sapere research group file:///C:/Users/smithmy/Downloads/Progress-Review-of-the-High-Performance-Manuka-Plantations-PGP-Programme-August-2017.pdf accessed December 11, 2017

McKee, M., R. Adany and D. Leon (2012); Illegally produced alcohol Is increasingly available in the UK and will add to alcohol's already great threat to public health; *BMJ 2012* 344:e1146 doi: 10.1136/bmj.e1146

MPI (2017) Manuka Honey http://www.mpi.govt.nz/growing-and-harvesting/honey-and-bees/manuka-honey/ accessed December 11, 2017

National Fraud Authority (2013); Annual Fraud Indicator https://www.gov.uk/government/uploads/system/uploads/attachment_data/file/206552/nfa-annual-fraud-indicator-2013.pdf accessed December 11, 2017

Newton, J. (2015); Inside the fake alcohol distillery: Plant for bottling counterfeit vodka raided as police seized 2,500 litres of fake wine and spirits http://www.dailymail.co.uk/news/article-2955934/Inside-fake-alcohol-distillery-Plant-bottling-counterfeit-vodka-raided-police-seized-2–500-litres-fake-wine-spirits.html accessed December 11, 2017

Oceana (2017); Seafood fraud and mislabelling in Ottawa; file:///C:/Users/smithmy/Downloads/http___www.oceana.ca_sites_default_files_ottawa_testing_report_en_final_0.pdf accessed December 11, 2017

O'Mahony, P.J. (2013); Finding horse meat in beef products—a global problem; *QJM: An International Journal of Medicine* 106(6):595–597,

Petrakis, E., L. Cagliani, P. Tarantilis, M. Polissiou and R. Consonni (2017); Sudan dyes in adulterated saffron (*Crocus sativus* L.): Identification and quantification by H NMR; *Food Chemistry* 217:418–24

Petrakis, E. and M. Polissiou (2017); Assessing saffron (*Crocus sativus* L.) adulteration with plant-derived adulterants by diffuse reflectance infrared Fourier transform spectroscopy coupled with chemometrics; *Talanta* 162:558–566

Pustjens, A.M., Y. Weesepoel and S. van Ruth (2016); Chapter 1: Food fraud and authenticity: Emerging issues and future trends; In: Innovation and Future Trends in Food Manufacturing and Supply Chain Technologies, pp. 3–20; ed. Craig Leadley http://dx.doi.org/10.1016/B978-1-78242-447-5.00001-0 accessed January 2, 2018

SSAFE (2017); Food Fraud Tool https://www.pwc.nl/en/industries/agrifood/ssafe-food-fraud-tool.html accessed December 15, 2017

Stone, D. and B. Heard (2010); VODKAT is not vodka: 'Extended' passing off extended; *Journal of Intellectual Property Law & Practice* 5(12):842–843

Tosun, M. (2013); Detection of adulteration in honey samples added various sugar syrups with 13C/12C isotope ratio analysis method; *Food Chemistry* 138:1629–1632

USAID (2008); Iraq a Strategy for Pomegranate http://pdf.usaid.gov/pdf_docs/Pnadp532.pdf accessed December 15 2017

Vanhaecke, L., W. Verbeke and H. De Brabander (2010); Glazing of frozen fish: Analytical and economic challenges; *Analytica Chimica Acta* 672:40–44

van Ruth, S.M., W. Huisman and P.A. Luning (2017); Food fraud vulnerability and its key factors; *Trends in Food Science & Technology* 67:70–75

van Uhm, D. and D. Siegel (2016); The illegal trade in black caviar; *Trends in Organized Crime* 19:67–87

Walker, M.J., M. Burns and D. Thorburn Burns (2013); Horse Meat in Beef Products – Species Substitution 2013; *Journal of the Association of Public Analysts* (Online) 41:67–106

Wei, G., J. Huang and J. Yang (2012); Safety standards and its impacts on China's honey export; *Journal of Integrative Agriculture* 11(4):684–693

Wong, E. and R. Hanner (2008; DNA barcoding detects market substitution in North American seafood; *Food Research International* 41:828–837

Worobiec, M. (2017); The road ahead for Northern California's wine Industry; Wine Spectator, October 25, 2017 http://www.winespectator.com/webfeature/show/id/California-Wine-Fire-Road-Ahead accessed December 15 2017

Index